AF332998

BORN INTO THIS WORLD

HEALTH ISSUES

PEDIATRICS, CHILD AND ADOLESCENT HEALTH

JOAV MERRICK – SERIES EDITOR –

NATIONAL INSTITUTE OF CHILD HEALTH AND HUMAN DEVELOPMENT, MINISTRY OF SOCIAL AFFAIRS, JERUSALEM

Positive Youth Development: Theory, Research and Application
Daniel TL Shek, Rachel CF Sun and Joav Merrick (Editors)
2012. ISBN: 978-1-62081-305-8
(Hardcover)

Tropical Pediatrics: A Public Health Concern of International Proportions
Richard R Roach, Donald E Greydanus, Dilip R Patel, Douglas N Homnick and Joav Merrick (Editors)
2012-September.
ISBN: 978-1-61942-831-7
(Hardcover)

Positive Youth Development: A New School Curriculum to Tackle Adolescent Developmental Issues
Hing Keung Ma, Daniel TL Shek and Joav Merrick (Editors)
2012- October. ISBN: 978-1-62081-384-3 (Hardcover)

Understanding Autism Spectrum Disorder: Current Research Aspects
Ditza A Zachor and Joav Merrick (Editors)
2012- November.
ISBN: 978-1-62081-353-9
(Hardcover)

Transition from Pediatric to Adult Medical Care
David Wood, John G Reiss, Maria E Ferris, Linda R Edwards and Joav Merrick (Editors)
2012- November.
ISBN: 978-1-62081-409-3
(Hardcover)

Child and Adolescent Health Yearbook 2012
Joav Merrick (Editor)
2012- November.
ISBN: 978-1-61942-788-4
(Hardcover)

Child Health and Human Development Yearbook 2011
Joav Merrick (Editor)
2012- December.
ISBN: 978-1-61942-969-7
(Hardcover)

Playing with Fire: Children, Adolescents and Firesetting
Hatim A Omar,
Carrie Howell Bowling and
Joav Merrick (Editors)
2013 - 4th Quarter.
ISBN: 978-1-62948-471-6
(Softcover)

School, Adolescence and Health Issues
Joav Merrick, Ariel Tenenbaum and
Hatim A Omar (Editors)
2014 - 1st Quarter. ISBN: 978-1-62948-702-1
(Hardcover)

Adolescence and Sexuality: International Perspectives
Joav Merrick, Ariel Tenenbaum and
Hatim A Omar (Editors)
2014 - 1st Quarter. ISBN: 978-1-62948-711-3
(Hardcover)

Child and Adolescent Health Yearbook 2013
Joav Merrick (Editor)
2014 - 2nd Quarter. ISBN: 978-1-63117-658-6
(Hardcover)

Adoption: The Search for a New Parenthood
Gary Diamond and Eva Arbel
(Authors)
2014 - 2nd Quarter. ISBN: 978-1-63117-710-1
(Hardcover)

Adolescence: Places and Spaces
Myra Taylor, Julie Ann Pooley and
Joav Merrick (Editors)
2014 - 2nd Quarter. ISBN: 978-1-63117-847-4
(Hardcover)

Pain Management Yearbook 2013
Joav Merrick (Editor)
2014 - 3rd Quarter. ISBN: 978-1-63117-944-0
(Hardcover)

Child Health and Human Development Yearbook 2013
Joav Merrick (Editor)
2014 - 3rd Quarter
ISBN: 978-1-63117-939-6
(Hardcover)

Born into this World: Health Issues
Donald E Greydanus,
Arthur N Feinberg and
Joav Merrick (Editors)
2014 - 3rd Quarter.
ISBN: 978-1-63321-667-9
(Hardcover)

PEDIATRICS, CHILD AND ADOLESCENT HEALTH

BORN INTO THIS WORLD

HEALTH ISSUES

DONALD E. GREYDANUS
ARTHUR N. FEINBERG
AND
JOAV MERRICK
EDITORS

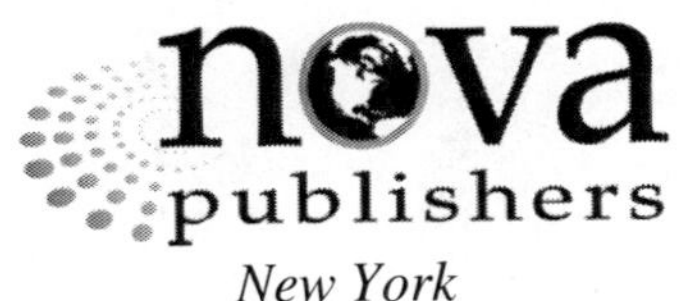

nova publishers
New York

NOTICE TO THE READER

The Publisher has taken reasonable care in the preparation of this book, but makes no expressed or implied warranty of any kind and assumes no responsibility for any errors or omissions. No liability is assumed for incidental or consequential damages in connection with or arising out of information contained in this book. The Publisher shall not be liable for any special, consequential, or exemplary damages resulting, in whole or in part, from the readers' use of, or reliance upon, this material. Any parts of this book based on government reports are so indicated and copyright is claimed for those parts to the extent applicable to compilations of such works.

Independent verification should be sought for any data, advice or recommendations contained in this book. In addition, no responsibility is assumed by the publisher for any injury and/or damage to persons or property arising from any methods, products, instructions, ideas or otherwise contained in this publication.

This publication is designed to provide accurate and authoritative information with regard to the subject matter covered herein. It is sold with the clear understanding that the Publisher is not engaged in rendering legal or any other professional services. If legal or any other expert assistance is required, the services of a competent person should be sought. FROM A DECLARATION OF PARTICIPANTS JOINTLY ADOPTED BY A COMMITTEE OF THE AMERICAN BAR ASSOCIATION AND A COMMITTEE OF PUBLISHERS.

Additional color graphics may be available in the e-book version of this book.

Library of Congress Cataloging-in-Publication Data

ISBN: 978-1-63321-667-9

Library of Congress Control Number: 2014945907

Published by Nova Science Publishers, Inc. † New York

CONTENTS

Introduction   **1**

Chapter 1   Born into this world - A historical view   **3**
                     Donald E Greydanus, MD, DrHC (Athens),
                     Arthur N Feinberg, MD, FAAP
                     and Joav Merrick, MD, MMedSc, DMSc

Section one: Issues in the newborn period   **17**

Chapter 2   Evaluation: During pregnancy, labor, delivery and of
                     the newborn   **19**
                     Arthur N Feinberg, MD, FAAP

Chapter 3   The late preterm newborn   **65**
                     Geoffrey De Tolve, MD

Chapter 4   Newborn screening   **83**
                     Arthur N Feinberg, MD, FAAP

Chapter 5   Resuscitation   **101**
                     Vinay N Reddy, MD

Chapter 6   Born premature: What does it mean?   **113**
                     I Leslie Rubin, MD

Chapter 7   Circumcision   **131**
                     Julian Wan, MD

Chapter 8   Environment and birth weight   **143**
                     Rebecca Ouyang

Chapter 9   Cycle of environmental health disparities   **157**
                     I Leslie Rubin, MD

Section Two: Acknowledgements   **175**

Chapter 10   About the editors   **177**

Chapter 11   About the Department of Pediatric and Adolescent
                        Medicine, Western Michigan University Homer
                        Stryker MD School of Medicine (WMED),
                        Kalamazoo, Michigan USA   **181**

Chapter 12   About the National Institute of Child Health and
                        Human Development in Israel   **185**

Chapter 13   About the book series "Pediatrics, child and
                        adolescent health"   **189**

Section Three: Index   **193**

Index   **195**

INTRODUCTION

In: Born into this World: Health Issues   ISBN: 978-1-63321-667-9
Editors: D. E. Greydanus, A. N. Feinberg et al.   © 2014 Nova Science Publishers, Inc.

Chapter 1

BORN INTO THIS WORLD - A HISTORICAL VIEW

Donald E Greydanus, MD, DrHC (Athens)[1],
Arthur N Feinberg, MD, FAAP[1]
and Joav Merrick, MD, MMedSc, DMSc[2,3,4,5,6]

[1]Department of Pediatric and Adolescent Medicine, Western Michigan
University Homer Stryker MD School of Medicine, Kalamazoo, Michigan,
United States
[2]National Institute of Child Health and Human Development, Jerusalem
Israel
[3]Office of the Medical Director, Health Services, Division for Intellectual
and Developmental Disabilities, Ministry of Social Affairs and Social
Services, Jerusalem, Israel
[4]Division of Pediatrics, Hadassah Hebrew University Medical Center, Mt
Scopus Campus, Jerusalem, Israel
[5]Kentucky Children's Hospital, University of Kentucky College of
Medicine, Lexington, Kentucky, United States
[6]Center for Healthy Development, School of Public Health, Georgia State
University, Atlanta, United States of America

---

* Correspondence: Professor Donald E Greydanus MD, Founding Chair, Department of Pediatric
and Adolescent Medicine, Western Michigan University Homer Stryker MD School of
Medicine, 1000 Oakland Drive, D48G, Kalamazoo, MI, 49008-1284, United States. E-mail:
Donald.Greydanus@med.wmich. org.

INTRODUCTION

Stéphane Tarnier (1828-1897) was the doyen of perinatology in France and as a Parisian obstetrician initiated principles of perinatal care that were further advanced by his students, Drs Budin and Pinard (1,2). The newborn could be called a real medical patient at the end of the 1800s when Professor Piérre-Constant Budin (1846-1907) provided newborns with hospital charts; he was director of the famous Pavilion des Debiles at the Maternité in Paris and is called by some the father of newborn medicine (3,4).

Professor Budin worked with the hospital's chief midwife, Madame Henry, and established a department of premature infants or "weaklings" that focused on three problems: temperature control, feeding, and correction of underlying disorders (5). He advocated the use of breastfeeding from the mother or a wet nurse and if the premature baby was not able to suck, milk was given via a spoon into the mouth or via a "nasal spoon" into the nose. The baby was weighed before and after the feeding and Professor Budin concluded that premature infants should take the amount of milk equivalent to or a little more than one-fifth of its body weight each day (5).

Also, Dr John William Ballantyne (Edinburgh obstetrician: 1861-1923) developed an overt master plan for maternal-fetal care continuity seeking to deal with the devastating effects of tuberculosis, typhoid fever, and syphilis (3). Another famous French obstetrician was Professor Adolphe Pinard (1844-1934) who was from Méry-sur-Seine and was an assistant to Professor Tarnier. Professor Pinard is considered a pioneer of modern perinatal care, taught infant care to pregnant women("puericulture movement"), and advocated for social care of indigent pregnant mothers as well as their babies while the mothers were pregnant and also after the birth (4,6). He established antenatal departments and wards in maternity hospitals in France (6).

The use of an incubator ("incubating cradle") for premature infants was first reported by French anatomist Jean Louis Paul Denucé (1824-1889) in 1857, one century after Ren? Antoine Ferchault De Réaumur (1683-1757), a French scientist known especially for his work in entomology, designed an egg incubator using a wood stove for its heat (4). A student of Professor Budin, Dr Martin A Couney (1870-1950), a German physician (identified by some as Coney), has been called the "incubator doctor" who brought this technology for premature and newborn infants to the United States in 1896 (7). Dr Couney conducted baby incubator exhibits in various places including the 1939-1940 New York World's Fair. In 1897 he published a letter to Lancet warning all to be aware of false purveyors of incubators by unprofessional persons (8).

Newborn care slowly but surely improved as ever more clinicians turned their attention to these "weakling." The German obstetrician, Carl Siegmund Franz Credé (1819-1892), introduced the use of 2% silver nitrate solution in the early 1880s to treat ophthalmia neonatorum; it became known as the Credéprophylaxis and was later reduced to 1% solution (8,9). The English orthopedic surgeon, William John Little, MD (1810-1894), identified an association between birth trauma and cerebral palsy—a condition previously blamed on complications of teething (10,11). Originally called cerebral paralysis by Dr Little in 1860 the current term was later popularized in 1887 by Sir William Osler, MD (1849-1919) the famous Canadian physician who became one of the four founding professors of Johns Hopkins hospital (12).

NEW BORN CARE ENTERS THE 20TH CENTURY

As the 1900s gave way to the 20th century, home deliveries gave way to hospital deliveries which led to increasing numbers of hospital nurseries and pediatricians becoming more directly involved in newborn care (13). Concern with infant mortality rates, child labor, and other negative issues affecting children led to the establishment of the Federal Children's Bureau on April 9, 1912 directed for 10 years by the American social reformer Julia Lathrop (1858-1932) to "...serve all children, to try to work out the standards of care and protection which should give to every child his fair chance in the world (14)."

The United States developed a birth registration process in 1915 for calculation infant mortality rates which dropped from over 180/1,000 live births in minority infants and 100/1,000 live births in white infants in 1915 to a rate of 6.05 in 2011 with continuing ethnic as well as racial disparities (13,15,16). A tug-of-war occurred for the newborn between the pediatrician and the obstetrician and Dr John Ballantyne (supra vida) noted that the newborn infant was in a "no-man's land" between these two fields (4). Gradually the pediatrician became more in charge of newborn care with the influence of pediatrician L Emmett Holt, MD who was author of the 1897 textbook (The diseases of infancy and childhood) as well as Julius Hess, MD who was chief of pediatrics at Michael Reese Hospital in Chicago, Illinois and developer of the Hess Incubator (4,7,17).

L Emmett Holt, MD (1855-1924) was Professor of Diseases of Children at New York Polyclinic and also the writer of another of his famous books "The care and feeding of children" in 1894. In addition, Professor Holt was

President of the American Association for the Study and Prevention of Infant Mortality and in 1913 noted: "We must eliminate the unfit by birth not by death. The race is to be most effectively improved by preventing marriage and reproduction of the unfit, among whom we would class the diseased, the degenerate, the defective, and the criminal (18)." Another but mayhaps more uplifting expert in feeding of children as well as children during this time was the German-American physician often credited being the father of Pediatrics in the US—Abraham Jacobi, MD (1830-1919) (19).

The US Sheppard Towner Maternity and Infancy Protection Act of 1921 was a law signed by President Warren Harding that promoted maternal and infant welfare--- including principles of infant care; it was developed by Julia Lathrop and other supporters of the American women's suffrage movement (4,20). Unfortunately the 1920s promoted some misconceptions about newborn care that included the removal of incubators, inappropriate use of water for regulation of newborn thirst, treatment of infant apnea using spirit of ammonia with whiskey, and other now archaic practices in newborn care (4). Newborn care improved in the 1930s with return of the incubator, use of the Hess box for oxygen delivery, improved hygiene, emphasis on lactation, and improved management for infection as well as diarrhea (4).

Progress in newborn care expanded in the decade of World War II with improvements in blood banking (due to American physician Charles Drew, MD [1904-1950]), fluid management, development of antibiotics (i.e., Sir Alexander Fleming, MD (1881-1955) and his discovery of penicillin in 1928 that was introduced in the 1940s), and emphasis on placement of pediatricians in the delivery room (4,21,22). Newborn care was stimulated by the 1941 finding of Australian ophthalmologist Sir Norman McAlister Gregg, MD (1982-1966) linking maternal rubella infection with congenital rubella syndrome (23).

Also monumental was the work of American pediatrician Louis K Diamond, MD (1902-1999), the father of Pediatric Hematology who, in 1942, noted the interconnection between the Rh factor and erythroblastosis which allowed this life-saving innovator to prevent kernicterus in most situations from 1946 onward by treatment with double volume exchange transfusion (4,24). Two decades later RhoGAM was utilized by New Zealand physician Sir William Liley (1929-1983) in 1963 demonstrating that it could be used to prevent erythroblastosis fetalis in newborns and infants.

We have witnessed the development of perinatal and neonatal medicine as it has developed over the past six decades since the use of RhoGam by Sir William Liley (25-27). The field of neonatology was identified with the publication of the inaugural book "Diseases of the newborn" by Alexander Schaeffer, MD (28). The field of pediatrics expanded to include pediatricians who cared for normal newborns and children but also those who specialized further to care for the sickest and smallest of newborns.

Gifted giants of pediatrics, as noted in the past, arose to take care of the newborn to further heights, as special care and intensive care units for newborns sprang up in the 1960s and a myriad of improvements emerged in ventilation as well as life support systems, fluid administration, infection control, and other key developments to prolong life in smaller and ever smaller human beings. These key, legendary pediatricians include Virginia Apgar, MD (1909-1974) with development of the Apgar score in 1953 (29-33), Mary Ellen Avery, MD (1927-2011) and her mentor Jeremiah Mead, MD (1920-2009) with research on surfactant deficiency (34,35), William A Silverman, MD (1917-2004) with research on retrolental fibroplasia (retinopathy of prematurity) as well as thermal temperature management (36-38), pediatric radiologist William H Northway Jr, MD's research on bronchopulmonary dysplasia (39), and Dr Tetsuro Fugiawara's research on surfactant administration, and so many, many more (4,40).

Certainly the advances made in care of the premature infant owe much to the research stimulated by the birth (at 32 weeks gestation) and death of President John F Kennedy's son, Patrick Bouvier Kennedy in 1963 (4). As advances in care of newborns in the neonatal intensive care unit (NICU) arose in the late 20th and now early 21st century, care in the normal newborn nursery has advanced as well. This book is inspired by this normal newborn unit and the health care personnel who provide expert care to the normal newborn. This book provides a summary of understanding of evaluation and management of normal late term and full term newborns.

THE FIRST BREATHS

The ancient Chinese emperor, Hwang-Ti (2698-2599 BCE) noted that death from respiratory failure was more commonly found in premature versus mature newborns—a concept also recorded in the Eber's Papyrus in ancient Egypt from 1500 BCE (41).

Getting air into the baby's nostrils was a concept from antiquity as illustrated by the above work of the Biblical prophet, Elisha (9th Century BCE), and also from this quote from the Babylonian Talmud (Talmud Bavli: 3rd -5th Centuries BCE):

"One may give a woman (about to give birth) all assistance possible... one may violate the Sabbath on her account … What is meant by "being of assistance"? … holding up the young, blowing air into its nostrils, and leading it to its mother's breast, so that it may suck."
Babylonian Talmud (translated by Michael L Rodkinson). Book I, Volume II, Chapter XVIII. Regulations regarding the clearing off of required space, the assistance to be given to cattle when giving birth to their young and to women about to be confined. Chapter XVIII, Page 282. 1903 (18).

The icons of early Western medicine, Hippocrates (460-380 BC) and Galen (129-199 AD) were aware of how placing a tube into the lungs of animals or humans and inserting air would lead to ventilation with rise of the chest (41). The fall of the Roman Civilization in the 5th century led to the loss of such knowledge for centuries as the Dark Ages descended on Europe. The great Persian physician, Avicenna (Ibn Sina) (980-1037 AD) described the process of intubation and reliable airway management---keeping this as well as many others facts of medicine alive allowing others in Europe and beyond to catch up centuries after his life with his famous "Book of healing and canon of medicine" (41,42).

A variety of methods have been utilized in the past with negative results and these include pinching, electrocution, hitting, use of raven's beak or corn cobs to dilate the newborn rectum, vigorous shaking, swinging, hanging upside down, holding the newborn in different positions, chest squeezing (Prochownich method), chest compression (Sylvester's method), cold water immersion (sometimes alternating with hot water immersion), brandy mist nebulization, tobacco smoke insufflated into the rectum, and others (41,43). Another method of improving respirations in newborns with depressed breathing was vigorous swinging of the newborn or stillborn called the Schultze's method or "schultzing" as developed by the German obstetrician, Bernhard Sigmund Schultze (1827-1919) (41,44,45).

"...give a small spoonful of pure wine into the neonate's mouth...[to] help the infant to regain its spirits when being agitated by the labors, which sometimes makes it so weak that it seems more dead than alive." (Bourgeois, 1609) (46)
"{The baby} should be rested on a warmed bed and brought near the fire, where the midwife having taken some wine into her mouth shall blow it into the infant's mouth, which can be repeated several times if necessary….She should warm all parts of the body to recall the blood and the spirits which retired during the weakness and endangered suffocation." (Mauriceau, mid-1600s) (46)

It was not until the 18th and 19th centuries that progress in resuscitation in the newborn was ignited by a variety of clinicians such as the Hunter, Chaussier, Gorcy and others (46,47). Perhaps the first pediatric airway was introduced by the English surgeon Benjamin Pugh (1715-1798) who developed his famed "air-pipe" at a time when fire place bellows were used to inflate dead or dying newborns with air (48,49).

"If the child does not breathe immediately upon Delivery, which sometimes it will not, especially when it has taken Air in the womb; wipe its Mouth, and press your Mouth to the Child's, at the same time pinching the Nose with your Thumb and Finger, to prevent air escaping; inflate the lungs; rubbing it before the Fire; by which method I have saved many." (Benjamin Pugh: English Surgeon: 1715-1798) (49)

The French obstetrician and anatomist, Francois Chaussier (1746-1828) introduced an air bag that was inflatable and attached to a mask or nostril tube and eventually containing a curved cannula for passage into the newborn's larynx. This advancement allowed resuscitation to occur with direct administration of air into the larynx and avoid introduction of soot/dust from the fireside bellows.

"There is one more means which sometimes works as by enchantment, it is to apply one's mouth on that of the infant and to blow into it, taking care to pinch the tip of the nose simultaneously. This method is so effective that it is really rare that others are useful if it fails." (Levret, 1766) (47)

The use of endotracheal intubation to resuscitate newborns may have initiated with Scheel in 1798 (50). Various clinicians were involved in resuscitation efforts of humans including newborns in the 18th and 19th centuries including the English physiologist and obstetrician, James Blundell (1790-1878) (51-56), the English surgeon John Hunter (1728-1793) (57,58), Scottish obstetrician William Hunter (1782), Ribemont, Pierre Budin, and others (44). For example, Ribemont (Alban Alphonse Ambroise Ribemont-Dessaignes [1847-1940]), a student of Tarnier, developed an improved endotracheal tube for newborns in 1877 while another Tarnier student, Budin, advocated endotracheal intubation of premature infants with depressed breathing (44).

In 1827 Leroy d'Etiolles (1798-1860) officiously lectured in Paris on a connection between ventilation and development of pneumothorax which resulted in a century of obdurate divagation and deliquescence of mouth-to-mouth as well as bellow air inflation and positive pressure ventilation in resuscitation efforts (41). This oratorical obfuscation also lead to the increased popularization of such resuscitation efforts as the Schultze swinglings or the Sylvester compression technique until the 1920s-1930s (44,46,59).

The number of reports discussing fetal termination via craniotomy or embryotomy were greater than reports discussing neonatal resuscitation efforts during this period into the second decade of the 20th century especially since caesarean sections were contraindicated if the mother had an infection (44). Successful resuscitation efforts for newborns were eventually seen due to a number of serendipitous factors, including increase in improved techniques, the ability to perform aseptic caesarean sections, and placing pediatricians in the delivery room (44).

Another improvement in resuscitation was the use of oxygen which had been tried as early as 1780, but gained more acceptance as part of newborn resuscitation techniques in the 20th century----though more research is needed on its precise use even today (59,60). Indeed various methods of air/oxygen delivery into airways and even the stomach were used since the early 1800s that were tried on stillborns until the 1950s (59).

The process of resuscitation (CPR) was improved in the 20th century with many successful innovations such as the Fell laryngoscope, Magill's intubation forceps, material that were not harmful to body tissues, tight-fitting endotracheal tubes, and improvement in CPR techniques as well as training of health care professionals (46,47,50,59-61). Modern ventilators were eventually developed in the 20th century stimulated by the poliomyelitis epidemics of this century (46). The 20th century witnessed improvement in adult and then pediatric resuscitation with the initiation of external defibrillation in 1956, mouth-to-mouth ventilation in CPR in 1958, and closed-chest compression in 1960 (61).

The 21st century is now marked by increased research to continuously refine these techniques with scientific evidence for which precise modus operandi are really well-founded (i.e., use of oxygen, meconium suctioning, hypothermia prevention), which ones are used only because of expert consensus (62,63), which ones are debated continuously by various "sages" (64-69), and what new knowledge awaits---knowledge that began in antediluvian times (41,50,70).

"Since intubation and positive pressure ventilation were first recommended... a pattern of resuscitation has evolved based on extrapolation and assumption rather than clinical measurement. There can be few areas of medicine where the potential benefit is so great but which have been subjected to so little evaluation" (Henderson, 1928) (71)

CONCLUSION

The mortality rate of newborns has been reduced in many parts of the world and we have learned much about how to keep more and more newborns alive especially when health care providers and society collaborate in this important endeavor and emphasize known preventative principles (72-76). We know that death of newborns causes emotional stress to the newborn's family as well as to the involved health caregivers (77). We are also learning about the historical rights of the fetus in modern society (78).

Current modern pediatric and perinatal treatments allow newborns in the current 21st century America to have a start on an overall life expectancy of 78.5 years (up to 76 years in males and 80.9 years in females) if they receive meticulous medical care even if born into a penurious state (79). Though we have learned much about caring for newborns, humans have also been killing their newborns since recorded time. Unfortunately this Kafkaesque killing continues based on many factors and female newborns remain at higher risk of gadarene murders than male infants even in the enlightened 21st century (80).

Our newborns must not be jeopardized by being considered as enfants terrible nor as feral golems but hailed as an answer to the statement of the auspicious American poet Joyce Kilmer (1886-1918):

"I think that I shall never see a poem as lovely as a tree…"

but of the things in life more lovely than a tree is the newborn! We do not need a Rube Goldberg machine to teach us how to care for newborns but qua the best imbued qualities in the Homo sapiens sapiens species, we need to simply love and care for these little beacons of our futurity. Indeed, newborns are a requisite, vatic aubade magnificently greeting our own dawn of existence in the complex, enigmatic circle of life that involves the living in the cosmos. The phrase "caring for the newborn" should be a utopic compendium of mutatis mutandis in the 21st century.

This elucidative disquisition is dedicated to giving these precious little ones a hortative, caring start to help them reach their full potential in the 21st century. We conclude that we should not kill them, but care for them to help them reach their full future in a troubled world. Even if we exist in a milieu that encourages such killing, we should resist it following the assuaging spirit of the expeditious Jewish midwives in ancient Egypt, Shifra (Shiphrah) and Puah, who refused to obey Pharaoh's disparaging decree to kill all Jewish newborn males in Exodus 1:15-20.

"The king of Egypt said to the Hebrew midwives, whose names were Shiphrah and Puah, 'When you are helping the Hebrew women during childbirth on the delivery stool, if you see that the baby is a boy, kill him; but if it is a girl, let her live.' The midwives, however, feared God and did not do what the king of Egypt had told them to do; they let the boys live" (Exodus 1:15-17)

REFERENCES

[1]   Dunn PM. Stéphane Tarnier (1828-1897), the architect of perinatology in France. Arch Dis Child Fetal Neonatal Ed 2002;86(2):F137-9.

[2]   Fraser M. Stéphane Tarnier and the origin of incubators for premature babies. Rep Proc Scott Soc Hist Med 1994-1996: 1-2.

[3]   Dunn PM. Professor Pierre Budin (1846-1907) of Paris, and modern perinatal care. Arch Dis Child Fetal Neonatal Ed 1995;73(3):F193-5

[4]   Lussky RC. A century of neonatal medicine. Minn Med 1999; 82: 1-8.

[5]   Budin P: Le Nourisson, Paris, Octave Doin, 1900 (English translation by Maloney WJ: The nursling. London: Caxton Publishing Co, 1907.

[6]   Dunn PM. Adolphe Pinard (1844-1934) of Paris and intrauterine paediatric care. Arch Dis Child Fetal Neonatal Ed 2006;91(3):F231-2.

[7]   Silverman WA. Incubator-baby slide shows. Pediatrics 1979;64(2): 127-41.

[8]   Schenkein S, Coney M. Infant incubators (letter-to-the-editor). Lancet 1897;2:744.

[9]   Dunn P. Dr. Carl Credé (1819-1892) and the prevention of ophthalmia neonatorum. Arch Dis Child Fetal Neonatal Ed 2000;83(2): F158-9.

[10]   Accardo P. William John Little and cerebral palsy in the nineteenth century. J Hist Med Allied Sci 1989;44(1):56-71.

[11]   Dunn PM. Dr. William Little (1810-1894) of London and cerebral palsy. Arch Dis Child Fetal Neonatal Ed 1995;72(3):F209-10.

[12]   Hansen AC. William Osler MD. J Natl Med Assoc 1986;78(10): 919.

[13]   Desmond MM. A review of newborn medicine in America: European past and guiding ideology. Am J Perinatol 1991;8(5):308-22.

[14]   URL: http://www.acf.hhs.gov/programs/cb/index.htm

[15]   MacDorman MF, Mathews TJ, Centers for Disease Control and Prevention (CDC). Infant deaths-United States, 2005-2008. MMWR Surveill Summ 2013;62(Suppl 3):171-5.

[16]   Lu MC, Johnson KA. Toward a national strategy on infant mortality. Am J Public Health 2014;104(Suppl 1): S13-6.

[17]   Dunn PM. Dr Emmett Holt (1855-1924) and the foundation of North American paediatrics. Arch Dis Child Fetal Neonatal Ed 2000;83(3): F221-3.

[18]   Meckel RA. Save the Babies: American Public Health Reform and the prevention of infant mortality, 1850-1929. Ann Arbor, MI: University of Michigan Press, 1998:118.

[19]   Ligon-Borden BL. Abraham Jacobi, MD: Father of American pediatrics and advocate for children's health. Semin Pediatr Infect Dis 2003;14(3): 246-9.

[20]   Kessler-Harris A. In pursuit of equity: Women, men, and the quest for economic citizenship in the Twenty-First Century America. New York: Oxford University Press, 2001.

[21]   Wilson BA, O'Connor WG, Willis MS. The legacy of Charles R. Drew MD, CM, MDSC. Immunohematology 2011;27(3):94-100.

[22]   Ligon BL. Sir Alexander Fleming: Scottish researcher who discovered penicillin. Semin Pediatr Infect Dis 2004;15(1):58-64.

[23]   Mackey DA. 2005 Gregg Lecture: Congenital cataracts—from rubella to genetics. Clin Experiment Opthalmol 2006;34(3):199-207.

[24]   Pearson CH. Replacement transfusion as a treatment of erythroblastosis fetalis, by Louis K. Diamond MD. Pediatrics 1948;2:520-524. Pediatrics 1998;102 (1 Pt 2):203-5.

[25]   Dunn PM. The birth of perinatal medicine in the United Kingdom. Semin Fetal Neonatal Med 2007;12(3):27-38.

[26]   Desmond MM. A review of newborn medicine in America: European past and guiding ideology. Am J Perinatol 1991;8(5):308-22.

[27]   Dudenhausen JW. 40 years of the Journal of Perinatal Medicine. J Perinatal Med 2013;41(1):3-4.

[28]   Schaffer AJ. Diseases of the newborn. Philadelphia, PA: Saunders, 1960.

[29]   Apgar V. Infant resuscitation, 1957. Conn Med 2007;71(9):553-5.

[30]   Galanakis E. Apgar score and Soranus of Ephesus. Lancet 1998; 352(9145):2012-3

[31]   Baskett TF. Virginia Apgar and the newborn Apgar score. Resuscitation 2000;47(3):215-7.

[32]   Appelgren L. The woman behind the Apgar score, Virginia Apgar. The woman behind the scoring system for quality control of the newborn. Läkartidningen 1991;88(14):1304-6.

[33]   Finster M, Wood M. The Apgar score has survived the test of time. Anesthesiology 2005;102(4):855-7.

[34]   Avery ME, Mead J. Surface properties in relation to atelectasis and hyaline membrane disease. AMA J Dis Child 1959;97(5 Pt 1):517-23.

[35]   Pincock P. Mary Ellen Avery. Lancet 2012;379(9816): 610.

[36]   Silverman WA. Compassion or opportunism? Pediatrics 2004;113(2): 402-3.

[37]   Watts G. William Silverman. BMJ 2005;330(7485): 257.

[38]   Oransky I. William Silverman. Lancet 2005;365(9454):116

[39]   Northway WHJr, Rosan RC, Porter DY. Pulmonary disease following respirator therapy of hyaline-membrane disease. Bronchopulmonary dysplasia. N Engl J Med 1967;276(7):357–68.

[40]   Fujiwara T, Chida S, Wataba Y, Maeta H, Morita T, Abe T. Artificial surfactant therapy in hyaline-membrane disease. Lancet 1980;315(8159):55-9.

[41]   O'Donnell CPF, Gibson AT, David PG. Pinching, electrocution, ravens' breaks, and positive pressure ventilation: a brief history of neonatal resuscitation. Arch Dis Child Fetal Neonatal Ed 2006;91(5): F369-73.

[42]   Khan A. Avicenna (Ibn Sina): Muslim physician and philosopher of the eleventh century. New York: Rosen Publishing Group, 2006.

[43]   Raju TN. History of neonatal resuscitation. Tales of heroism and desperation. Clin Perinatol 1999;26(3):629-40.

[44]   Rubin LP. Abstract. The development of newborn resuscitation in Europe and North America from the 18th to early 20th centuries. Pediatric Res 1998;43:118.

[45]   Baskett TF, Nagele F. Bernhard Schultze and the swinging neonate. Resuscitation 2001;51(1):3-6.

[46]   Obladen M. History of neonatal resuscitation. Part 1: Artificial ventilation. Neonatology 2008;94(3):144-9.

[47]   Zaichkin J, Wiswell TE. The history of neonatal resuscitation. Neonatal Netw 2002; 21(5): 21-8.

[48]   Basket TF. The resuscitation greats. Benjamin Pugh: the air-pipe and neonatal resuscitation. Resuscitation 2000;44(3):153-5.

[49]   Wilkinson DJ. Benjamin Pugh and his air-pipe. In: Marshall Barr A, Boulton T, Wilkinson DJ, eds. Essays on the history of anaesthesia: Selected and revised contributions by members of the History of Anaesthesia Society series 1, 1986-1989. London: Royal Society of Medicine Press, 1996.

[50]   Obladen M. History of neonatal resuscitation-part 3: endotracheal intubation. Neonatology 2009;95(3):198-202.

[51]   Blundell J. Dr. Blundell's reason for his retirement from the Medical School of Guy's Hospital. Lancet 1834-5;i:28.

[52]   Young JH. James Blundell (1790-1878) Experimental physiologist and obstetrician. Med Hist 1964;8(2):159-69.

[53]   No authors. James Blundell (1790-1877) physiologist and obstetrician. JAMA 1968;204(9):822-3.

[54]   Sørensen T. James Blundell, 27 December 1790-15 January 1878. Professor of physiology and obstetrics at Guy's Hospital 1823-1834. Ugeskr Laeger 1983;145 Spec No:5-49. [Danish]

[55]   Welck M, Borg P, Ellis H. James Blundell MD Edin FRCP (1790-1877): pioneer of blood transfusion. J Med Biogr 2010;18(4):194-7.

[56]   Dunn PM. Dr. James Blundell (1790-1878) and neonatal resuscitation. Arch Dis Child 1989;64(4 Spec No):494-5.

[57]   Moore W. The knife man: The extraordinary life and times of James Hunter, father of modern survery. New York: Crown Publishing Group, 2005.

[58]   Toledo-Pereyra LH. Birth of scientific surgery. John Hunter versus Joseph Lister as the father or founder of scientific surgery. J Invest Surg 2010;23(1):6-11.

[59]   Cataldi L, Fanos V. Neonatal resuscitation: a fascinating story! Acta Biomed Ateneo Parmense 2000;71(Suppl 1):671-2.

[60]   Obladen M. History of neonatal resuscitation. Part 2: oxygen and other drugs. Neonatology 2009;95(1):91-6.

[61]   Paraskos JA. History of CPR and the role of the national conference. Ann Emerg Med 1993;22(2 Pt 2):275-80.

[62]   Kattwinkel J, Niermeyer S, Nadkami V, Tibballs J, Phillips B, Ziderman D et al. Resuscitation of the newly born infant: an advisory statement from the Pediatric Working Group of the International Liaison Committee on Resuscitation. Resuscitation 1999;40(2:710-88.

[63]   International Liaison Committee on Resuscitation. The International Liaison Committee on Resuscitation (ILCOR) consensus on science with treatment recommendations for pediatric and neonatal patients: pediatric basic and advanced life support. Pediatrics 2006;117(5):e955- 77.

[64]   Escobedo M. Moving from experience to evidence: changes in the US Neonatal Resuscitation Program based on International Liaison Committee on Resuscitation Review. J Perinatol 2008;28(Suppl 1): S35-40.

[65]   Raghuveer TS, Cox AJ. Neonatal resuscitation: an update. Am Fam Physician 2011;83(8):911-8.

[66]   Davis PG, Dawson JA. New concepts in neonatal resuscitation. Curr Opin Pediatr 2012;24(2):147-53.

[67]   O'Donnell CP. Turn and face the strange-ch..ch..ch..changes to neonatal resuscitation guidelines in the past decade. J Paediatr Child Health 2012; 48(9):735-9.

[68]   Wyckoff MH. Neonatal resuscitation guidelines versus the reality of the delivery room. J Pediatr 2013;163(6):1542-3.

[69]   McCarthy LK, Morley CJ, Davis PG, Kamlin CO, O'Donnell CP. Timing of interventions in the delivery room: does reality compare with neonatal resuscitation guidelines. J Pediatr 2013;163(6): 553-1557.e1.

[70]   Nightengale B. A lifetime of "firsts". Adv Neonatal Care 2009;9(5): 259-51.

[71]   Henderson Y. The prevention and treatment of asphyxia in the newborn. JAMA 1928;90:583-6.

[72]   Souza J, WHO Multicountry Survey on Maternal and Newborn Health Research Network. The World Health Organization Multicountry Survey on Maternal and Newborn Health project at a glance: the power of collaboration. BJOG 2014;121(Suppl 1):v-viii.

[73]   Vogel J, Souza J, Mori R, Morisaki N, Lumbiganon P, Laopaiboon M et al. Maternal complications and perinatal mortality: findings of the The World Health Organization Multicountry Survey on Maternal and Newborn Health. BJOG 2014;121(Suppl 1):76-88.

[74]   Ganchimeg T, Ota E, Morisaki N, Laopaiboon M, Lumbignon P, Zhang J et al. Pregnancy and childbirth outcomes among adolescent mothers: a World Health Organization multicountry study. BJOG 2014;121(Suppl 1):40-8.

[75]   Linderkamp O, Gharavi B, Schott C. The concept of tender care of premature infants: A review. Kinderkrankenschwester 2004;23(8): 312-6.

[76]   Singh M. The art, science and philosophy of newborn care. Indian J Pediatr 2014 Mar 19. EPub ahead of print.

[77]   Ben-Ezra M, Palgi Y, Walker R, Many A, Hamam-Raz Y. The impact of perinatal death on obstetrics nurses: a longitudinal and cross-sectional examination. J Perinat Med 2014;42(1):75-81.

[78]   Harrison MR. Unborn: historical perspectives of the fetus as a patient. Pharos Alpha Omega Alpha Honor Med Soc 1982;45(1):19-24.

[79]   United States life tables, 2009. URL: http://www.cdc.gov/nchs/data/nvsr/nvsr62/nvsr62_07.pdf.

[80]   Carter J. A call to action: Women, religion, violence, and power. New York: Simon Schuster, 2014.

SECTION ONE: ISSUES IN THE NEWBORN PERIOD

In: Born into this World: Health Issues
Editors: D. E. Greydanus, A. N. Feinberg et al.

ISBN: 978-1-63321-667-9
© 2014 Nova Science Publishers, Inc.

Chapter 2

EVALUATION: DURING PREGNANCY, LABOR, DELIVERY AND OF THE NEWBORN

Arthur N Feinberg[*], *MD, FAAP*

Department of Pediatric and Adolescent Medicine, Western Michigan
University Homer Stryker MD School of Medicine, Kalamazoo, Michigan,
United States of America

The overall goal of this review is to enhance knowledge and skills for health providers in the newborn nursery. We present a systematic approach starting with a good prenatal history (maternal health and personal-social) and gestational history along with a systematic scheme for a thorough newborn assessment including physical examination and pre and post-natal objective testing. We emphasize the importance of monitoring and discuss several problems that may affect a term newborn, specifically growth problems, large-for-gestational age (LGA) and small for gestational age (SGA), temperature instability (hyper/hypothermia), tachypnea and apnea, vomiting, lethargy/poor feeding, irritability/ jitteriness, seizures, pallor/plethora, cyanosis, heart murmurs jaundice, and dermatologic conditions. The ultimate goal is for the health provider to acquire a strong fund of knowledge and to develop advancing skills in using this knowledge in diagnosis and management of these problems.

---

[*] Correspondence: Professor Arthur N Feinberg, MD, Department of Pediatric and Adolescent Medicine, Western Michigan University Homer Stryker MD School of Medicine, 1000 Oakland Drive, D48G, Kalamazoo, MI 49008-1284 United States. E-mail: arthur.feinberg@med.wmich.edu.

INTRODUCTION

The goals of this review are:

- To develop a prenatal history encompassing early, mid and late pregnancy, and delivery. We will emphasize maternal medical, family and social history, monitoring for prenatal diagnosis and fetal monitoring at labor and delivery.
- To review a thorough normal newborn assessment. We examine by region and evaluate each for inspection, palpation, percussion and auscultation where applicable.
- To discuss usual monitoring of normal term newborns.
- To present key post natal problems as reported by a caretaker or health professional.
- To develop a basic clinical approach to the most common problems in the newborn period, defined as the first 30 days of life: growth problems, large-for-gestational age (LGA) and small for gestational age (SGA), temperature instability (hyper/hypothermia), tachypnea and apnea, vomiting, lethargy/poor feeding, irritability/jitteriness, seizures, pallor/plethora, cyanosis, heart murmurs jaundice, and dermatologic conditions. Please refer to subsequent chapters to build upon the initial information provided herein.

PRENATAL HISTORY

Maternal problems

Infectious: Gather a thorough history on any maternal infectious illness during the pregnancy. Most likely the mother was screened for Group B streptococcal infection. If she was positive, was she treated adequately with antibiotics during labor (doses every 4 hours with last dose within 4 hours of delivery)? Were there any exposures to other bacteria such as E Coli (maternal urinary tract infection), listeria or tuberculosis? Did mother have any sexually-transmitted infections such as syphilis, gonorrhea, human immunodeficiency virus (HIV), chlamydia or ureaplasma? Viral infections during early pregnancy such as rubella, cytomegalovirus, varicella will cause fetal malformations. Hepatitis B and C will cause disease in newborns due to maternal transmission. Herpes simplex types 1 and 2 may produce a sepsis-like picture and can be overwhelming and devastating. Also, Enterovirus will cause a sepsis-like picture with jaundice, myocarditis or meningitis. Parasitic infestations, specifically toxoplasmosis will also cause fetal anomalies. A careful travel history will help elucidate possible exposures to other parasites.

Table 1. Non-infectious maternal conditions affecting the newborn (Adapted from Nelson Textbook of Pediatrics, 17th Edition, WB Saunders, 2004)

Maternal Condition	Newborn Findings
Congenital Heart Disease	Intrauterine Growth Retardation (IUGR)
Diabetes Mellitus	Hypoglycemia, hypocalcemia, polycythemia, large-for-gestational age, LGA, microcolon, asymmetric septal hypertrophy, caudal regression syndrome
Hypertension	IUGR
Obesity	Macrosomia, Hypoglycemia
Hyperthyroidism	Transient neonatal thyrotoxicosis
Hypothyroidism	Neonatal hypothyroidism
Hyperparathyroidism	Neonatal hypocalcemia
Immune thrombocytopenic purp	Neonatal thrombocytopenia
Myasthenia gravis	Transient weakness
Malignancy	Metastasis, fetal effects of treatment
Sickle cell anemia	IUGR
Systemic Lupus Erythematosus	Rash anemia, thrombocytopenia, neutropenia, 3° heart block
Renal failure	IUGR
Seizure disorder	Fetal effects of medications (see Table 3)

Non-infectious: Maternal medical history is important. Ask about common conditions such as diabetes mellitus, hypertension, endocrinological disorders such as hypo/hyperthyroisism, maternal immunological disorders that predispose to antibody transmission across the placenta (immune thrombocytopenic purpura, myasthenia gravis, collagen-vascular disorders et al), as they have profound effects on newborns. Maternal pulmonary cardiac, renal, hematological/oncological and neurological disorders may play a role in newborn outcome as will many of the medications used to treat these conditions. Are there any potentially inheritable conditions?

It is critical to obtain a full environmental and social history. Is the fetus at risk because of homelessness or unsanitary surroundings? Does the mother have a history of substance abuse including tobacco, alcohol or street drugs? Was there exposure to environmental hazards such as chemicals or pesticides?

Evaluate any medication the mother took during the pregnancy for any effect on the fetus or newborn infant, either teratogenic or symptomatic. See tables 1-3 below for maternal conditions and fetal exposures that are problematic (1).

Table 2. Infectious maternal conditions and their fetal effects (Adapted from Nelson Textbook of Pediatrics, 17th Edition, WB Saunders, 2004)

Maternal Condition	Newborn findings
Bacterial	
Group B streptococcus	Sepsis, pneumonia, meningitis
E Coli	Sepsis, pneumonia, meningitis
Klebsiella, Proteus,	Sepsis, pneumonia, meningitis
Pseudomonas	Sepsis, pneumonia, meningitis, conjunctivitis
Neisseria gonorrhoeae	(ophthalmia)
Mycoplasma pneumoniae	Pneumonia
Chlamydia trachomatis	Conjunctivitis
Syphilis	Snuffles, rhagades, saddle-nose deformity, metaphysitis, jaundice, hepatosplenomegaly (HSM)
Viral	
Rubella	IUGR, Cataracts, microphthalmia, HSM, Pulmonic Stenosis, Patent ductus, deafness, "blueberry muffin" skin (thrombocytopenia)
Varicella	
Embryopathy	Cicatrix scarring, poor limb development, multiple eye, brain and spinal cord abnormalities
Perinatal disease	Severe chickenpox, pneumonia, hepatitis, encephalitis
Cytomegalovirus (CMV)	
Embryopathy	IUGR, HSM, jaundice, purpura, microcephaly, cerebral calcifications, chorioretinitis, deafness.
Perinatal disease	Pneumonia, sepsis-like picture
Herpes Hominis	SEM (skin-eye mucous membrane), encephalitis, systemic (hepatic)
Hepatitis B, C	Neonatal Hepatitis B, C infection
Parvovirus B 19	Anemia, fetal hydrops
Enterovirus (Echo-Coxsakie)	Sepsis-picture, jaundice, myocarditis, meningitis
Parasitic	
Toxoplasmosis (embryopathy)	Similar to CMV + hydrocephalus

PRENATAL TESTING

Modern prenatal care involves monitoring for many potential problems. By time of delivery, maternal blood type, group B strep, rubella, hepatitis and possibly HIV status are documented on the chart, all of with which the pediatrician should be familiar. Alpha Fetoprotein levels will be elevated in neural tube defects, gastroschisis/omphalocoele, cystic hygroma multiple gestation and congenital nephrosis; it will be diminished in trisomies and intrauterine growth retardation (IUGR). All pregnant women are monitored for any conditions they may have (e.g., anemia, diabetes) in order to allow for best fetal outcomes.

Ultrasonography has become routine for almost all pregnancies and is most helpful in prenatal diagnosis and monitoring fetal growth. Normal intrauterine growth patterns are well-established and appear in figure 1 below. Oligohydramnios and polyhydramnios have many serious implications for a fetus and ultrasound easily identifies them (see table 4 below). Many anatomic defects detected before birth allow for appropriate anticipation on the part of both family and physician, and in some cases, pre-natal therapy. Detectable anatomic conditions are spina bifida, hydrocephalus, agenesis of the corpus callosum, Dandy-Walker malformation, hydronephrosis, omphalocoele/gastroschisis, gastrointestinal obstruction and diaphragmatic hernia. Nuchal pad thickening occurs in Turner syndrome and trisomies 21 and 18.

Table 3. Teratogenic effects of maternal exposures during pregnancy (Adapted from Nelson Textbook of Pediatrics, 17th Edition, WB Saunders, 2004)

Agent	Effect
Anti-cancer drugs	Fetal loss, malformations (aminopterin, cytoxan, azathioprine, 6MP)
Busulfan	IUGR, cleft palate,multiple endocrine gland abnormalities
Antibiotics	
Aminoglycosides	Deafness
Tetracyclines	Hypoplastic teeth, cataract, limb malformations
Chloroquine	Hearing loss
Quinine	Abortion, thrombocytopenia, deafness
Nitrofurantoin	Hemolytic anemia in pts with G6PD
Cephalosporins	Direct + Coombs test
Sulfonamides	Interfere with bilirubin protein binding, hemolysis in G6PD pts

Table 3. (Continued)

Anti-seizure medications	
Carbamazepine	
Phenytoin	Spina bifida
Valproate	↑ fontanel, hypertelorism, facial cleft, hypoplastic nails, low hairline
Trimethadione	Midface hypopolasia, narrow bi-frontal diameter, cardiac lesions, hyperconvex nails
Phenobarbital	Midface hypoplasia, prominent forehead, up-slanted eyebrows, short up-turned nose, midline cardiac defects, genital anomalies
	Vitamin K deficiency, sedation
Anti-inflammatory drugs	
Salicylates	
Ibuprofen	Bleeding, prolonged gestation
Indomethacin	Oligohydramnios, pulmonary hypertension
	Oligria, oligohydramnios, pulm hypertension, intestinal perforation
Antihypertensive drugs	
Atenolol	
Propranolol	IUGR, hypoglycemia
Reserpine	Hypoglycemia, bradycardia, apnea
Captopril	Stuffy nose, drowsiness, hypo/hyperthermia
	Oligohydramnios, ↓renal function
Steroid medications	
Progesterones, anabolic steroids	Fetal masculinization
Prednisone	Oral clefts
Thyroid medications	
Iodide	Goiter
Methimazole, Propothiouracil	Goiter, hypothyroidism
Diuretics	
Acetazolamide	
Thiazades	Metabolic acidosis
Vitamin D	Thrombocytopenia
Isotretinoin (Accutane)	Hypercalcemia, supravalvular aortic stenosis
	Multiple facial, skeletal and cardiac anomalies
Psychotropic drugs	
Thalidomide	
Lithium	Phocomelia, deafness
Haliperidol	Ebstein's anomaly
Imipramine	Withdrawal
Fluoxetine	Withdrawal
	Withdrawal, hypertonicity
Environmental toxins	
Hypertheremia	
Mercury	Spina bifida

Polychlorinated biphenyls (PCB)	Deafness, blindness, peripheral neuropathy (Minimata disease) IUGR, skin lesions
Anticoagulant Coumadin	Vitamin K deficiency, bleeding, hypoplastic nose, bone stippling, seizures
Drugs of Abuse Cocaine Amphetamines Opiates Tobacco	IUGR, microcephaly, gastroschisis, seizures Congenital heart lesions, withdrawal syndrome Withdrawal syndrome IUGR, sudden infant death syndrome
Medications used during labor Dexamethasone Oxytocin Magnesium Sulfate Sympathomimetic tocolytics	Periventricular leukomalacia Jaundice, hyponatremia Respiratory depression, lethargy, meconium plug tachycardia

Table 4. Etiologies of Oligohydramnios and Polyhydramnios (Adapted from Nelson Textbook of Pediatrics, 17th Edition, WB Saunders, 2004)

Oligohydramnios	Polyhydramnios
IUGR Amniotic fluid leak Anuria (renal agnesis, obstruction) Twin-twin transfusion Meds (ACE inhibitors, Inndomethacin)	Anencephaly-hydrancephaly-hydrocephaly Upper GI obstruction (duodenal atresia, et al) Diaphragmatic hernia Cystic adenomatoid malformation of lung Trisomies TORCH infections Fetal hydrops immune, non-immune Maternal diabetes, twin-twin transfusion (recipient), polyuria, chylothorax, teratoma

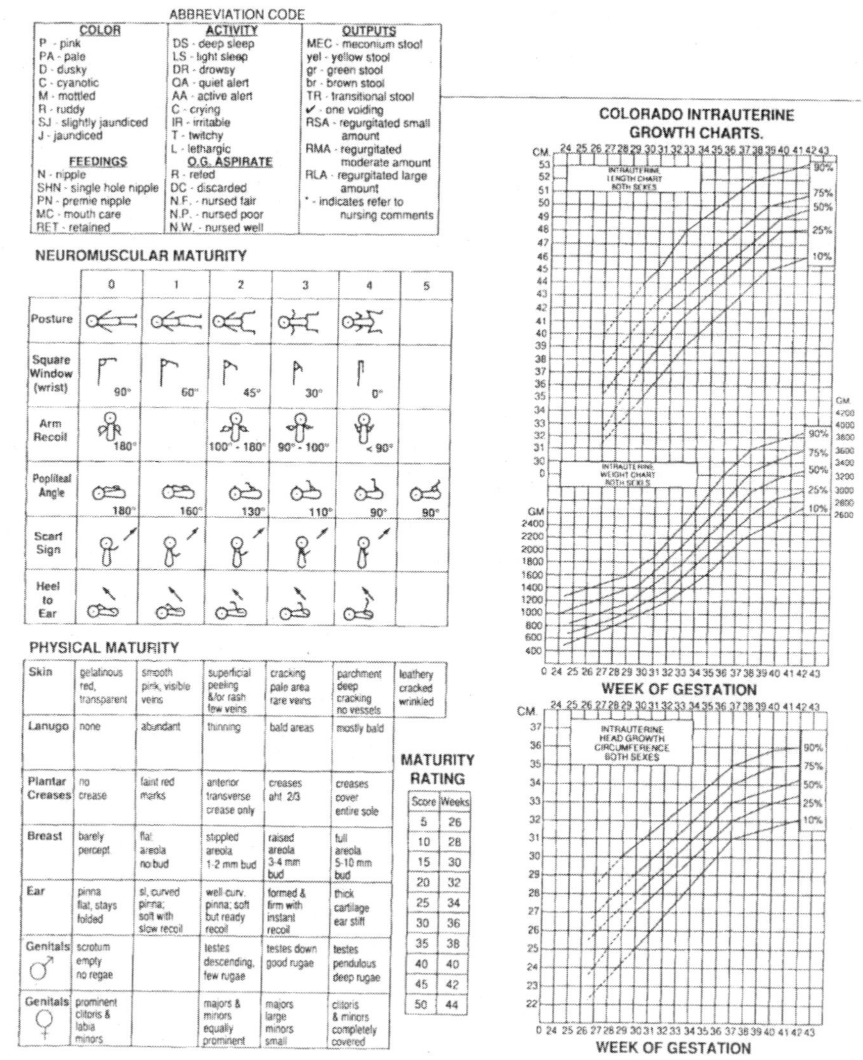

Figure 1. Evaluation of length, weight, head circumference and gestational age.

Measuring the distance from the skull to the uterine wall determines scalp edema that may be present in fetal hydrops.

Fetal cardiac monitoring may reveal potentially treatable arrhythmias such as supraventricular tachycardia and heart block.

Amniocentesis has many helpful applications during gestation, specifically, to evaluate chromosomes of a fetus in high risk situations such as family history or advanced maternal age. Assays for amino acids, organic acids, hormones and enzymes are helpful for diagnosing metabolic disorders prenatally. Amniotic fluid is helpful for following pregnancies with Rh isoimmunization (optical density) and determining fetal lung maturity (lecithin/sphingomyelin ratio). Cordocentesis obtains fetal blood which provides information regarding hematologic and infectious conditions (2,3).

MONITORING PREGNANCY, LABOR AND DELIVERY

It is important to assess and maintain placental sufficiency during gestation. Non-stress tests (NSTs), contraction stress tests (CSTs) and biophysical profiles (BFPs) measure fetal well-being, a reflection of placental sufficiency. NSTs assess fetal heart rate increases associated with normal movement. CSTs assess the fetal heart rate during uterine contractions, either spontaneous, or induced by nipple massage or oxytocin administration. The BFP measures fetal heart rate, breathing, tone and movement along with amniotic fluid volume.

During labor, fetal monitoring assesses changes in heart rate associated with uterine contractions. Early decelerations are due to head compression and are common and benign. Variable decelerations are a consequence of cord compression and may be ominous. Late decelerations result from fetal hypoxia due to uterine vessel spasm and indicate the need for immediate delivery. Beat-to-beat variability is also an indicator of fetal well-being, the loss of which is ominous. A steady, unvarying heart rate usually indicates catecholamine production as a consequence of significant fetal hypoxia and distress. The pediatrician should be aware of any abnormalities of these studies in their newborns, particularly if they are attending a delivery (3). Personnel trained and qualified in neonatal resuscitation should be present at all deliveries (4).

THE NEWBORN ASSESSMENT

Gestalt: Initial impression can be most useful in determining which infants need extra attention. Assess overall state of arousal by evaluating whether the newborn is asleep (deeply or lightly); awake with small amount of movement, awake with significant movement or crying. Is the cry lusty, or is it weak or high-pitched? Is the baby consolable? Assess newborn color and respiratory effort. Is the baby blue, or pink? Is he/she breathing comfortable? If it is rapid, is it quiet or noisy? Is the breathing rate too slow, or are there periods of apnea? How is the infant's posture? Normally a term newborn will assume flexion of all extremities, except for the thighs which abduct (see figures 2a and 2b). Are there any obvious malformations on immediate observation? Refer to the chapter on dysmorphology for more details.

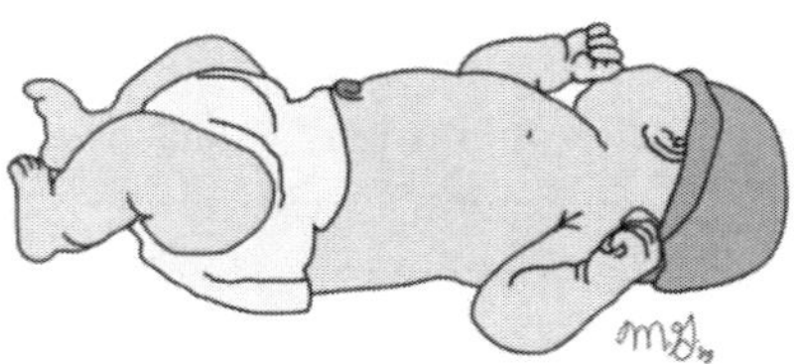

Figure 2a. Normal newborn posture.

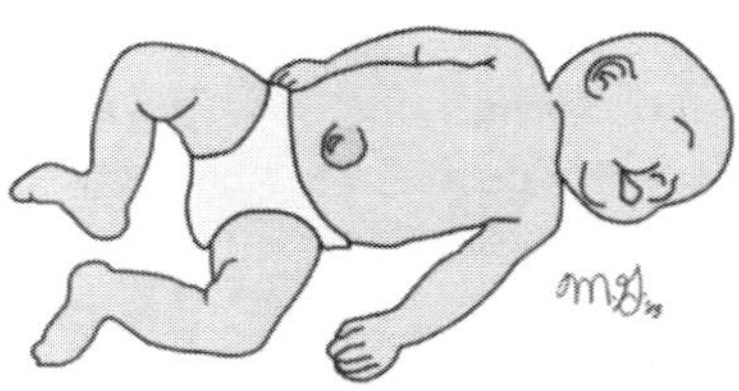

Figure 2b.Hypotonic newborn posture.

The Apgar score: Immediately upon delivery assess the newborn by the standard Apgar score as illustrated in table 5. Usually hospital personnel will perform this evaluation at age 1 minute and 5 minutes. If the score is <7, the evaluation is repeated every 5 minutes up to 20 minutes or two scores of ≥7, whichever comes first. If heart rates and respirations are extremely low it will be necessary to perform appropriate neonatal resuscitation.

Transition: Newborn transition from fetal to neonatal life usually takes a few hours and reflects itself in changes in color, pulse, respiration, alertness and activity, similar to the Apgar score. A normal newborn may appear slate-blue initially, but will become pink to ruddy during the transition period. Also, tachypnea to levels of 60-100 breaths/min will occur during the first hour, possibly due to amniotic fluid accumulated in the lung or as a correction for initial metabolic acidosis. Normally a newborn is awake and active with good tone during the first 60 minutes of life, and then may sleep afterwards.

Table 5. Apgar score for newborn assessment (From Fletcher, Physical Diagnosis in Neonatology, Lippincott-Raven 1998)

Sign	0	1	2
Heart rate	Absent	<100 bpm	>100 bpm
Respirations	Absent	Weak cry, hypoventilation	
Muscle tone	Limp	Some flexion	Active motion
Reflex irritability	No response	Grimace	Cough or sneeze
Color	Blue or pale	Pink, acrocyanosis	Completely pink

Measurements: For a term newborn, small for gestational age falls two standard deviations the mean of 3,175 gm (7#) at ,2500 grams (5# 8 oz), and large for gestational age falls 2 SD above the mean at 4,000 grams (8# 13 oz.). Neonatal length, weight and head circumference are plotted in figure 1. Although these are the standard measurements, take others if clinically necessary. Some of these are head measurements such as occipital/frontal diameter and fontanelle size, ocular measurements such as outer and inner canthal distance, palpebral fissure slant and corneal diameter, ear measurements such as position, rotation, and size, mouth measurements such as (columella and philtrum), chest measurements such as thoracic circumference, internipple distance and sternal length, and perineal measurements such as anal placement, penile length and testicular volume.

Gestational age: The new Ballard score assesses gestational age (see figure 1). Although term gestation is defined as 37-42 weeks, much new information has been forthcoming regarding the late pre-term infant (34-36 6/7 weeks). Please consult the chapter later in the book on this newly emerging topic. After 40 weeks gestation the fetus will often lose weight in-utero even to the point as to be considered small for gestation al age (SGA).They may be subject to asphyxia, hypoglycemia and polycythemia (5). Large for gestational age (LGA) babies often have immediate problems to address such as birth injury (ecchymosis, intracranial hemorrhage, clavicle fracture, diaphragmatic and brachial plexus paralysis). Metabolic problems may include jaundice, hypoglycemia, hyperviscosity syndrome, renal vein thrombosis and seizures. Etiologies for LGA babies include maternal diabetes, obesity, and chromosomal syndromes such as Beckwith-Weidemann and cerebral gigantism (Sotos syndrome). Small for gestational age babies are usually secondary to placental insufficiency from infection, infarction malformation, tumor or twin-to-twin transfusion. Maternal conditions such as hypertension (toxemia, placental abruption or HELLP syndrome), or renal disease, malnutrition and lack of prenatal care contribute toward poor fetal growth. Primary fetal conditions, most commonly chromosomal disorders congenital anomalies infection and immunodeficiency are causes of poor intrauterine growth. Small for gestational age infants will often have problems with hypoxia, acidosis, hypoglycemia and polycythemia.

Infant Name: _______________ MRN# _______________

Maternal History

Mom's Name _______________ Age _____ Type/RH _____ HBSA: ☐ Pos ☐ Neg

OB. Doctor _______________ G _____ P _____ AB _____ LC _____ RPR: ☐ Pos ☐ Neg

Prenatal History _______________ EDC _____ Rubella: ☐ Immune ☐ Non Immune

AROM/SROM _____ Date/Time _______________ Hrs. _______________ HIV: ☐ Pos ☐ Neg ☐ Declined ☐ Pending

GBBS: ☐ Pos ☐ Neg ☐ Unknown Treated in Labor greater than 4 hours ☐ Yes ☐ No ☐ Antibiotic: _______________

Complications: During Labor _______________

During Delivery _______________

Type of Delivery: Meds Prior to Delivery: _______________

☐ Vaginal ☐ C-Section _______________ Physician: _______________

Infant History

Birthdate _______________ Time _______________ Apgars: 1 min _____ 5 min. _____ Physician After Discharge: _______________

Delivery Complications _______________

Sex ☐ M ☐ F Wt. _____ LBS _____ OZ _____ GMS. _____ % TILE LENGTH: _____ IN _____ CM _____ %TILE

E.G.A.: BY DATES: _____ WKS. By DUBOWITZ: _____ WKS. HC: _____ IN _____ CM _____ %TILE

☐ Breast ☐ Bottle

PHYSICIAN ADMITTING AND DISCHARGE PHYSICAL

ADM. PHYSICAL DATA

(Code: ☑ = No abnormalities ⬭Circle⬭ = Abnormalities present)

1 ☐ Reflexes	7 ☐ Lungs	12 ☐ Anus
2 ☐ Skin: color, lesions	8 ☐ Heart	13 ☐ Trunk/Spine
3 ☐ Head/Neck	9 ☐ Abdomen	14 ☐ Extremities/Joints
4 ☐ Eyes	10 ☐ Umbilicus	15 ☐ Tone/Appearance
5 ☐ ENT	11 ☐ Genitals	16 ☐ Femoral pulses
6 ☐ Thorax		

DISCHARGE PHYSICAL DATA

(Code: ☑ = No abnormalities ⬭Circle⬭ = Abnormalities present)

1 ☐ Reflexes	7 ☐ Lungs	12 ☐ Anus
2 ☐ Skin: color, lesions	8 ☐ Heart	13 ☐ Trunk/spine
3 ☐ Head/Neck	9 ☐ Abdomen	14 ☐ Extremities/Joints
4 ☐ Eyes	10 ☐ Umbilicus	15 ☐ Tone/Appearance
5 ☐ ENT	11 ☐ Genitals	16 ☐ Femoral pulses
6 ☐ Thorax		

☐ EARLY DISCHARGE/SINGLE EXAM PERFORMED

DESCRIPTION OF ABNORMAL FINDINGS (if any)

DISCHARGE SUMMARY ☐ Normal Course ☐ Other: _______________

Wt. _______________ HEAD CIRCUM _______________

DATE _____ Signature: _______________ | DATE _____ Signature: _______________

Hepatitis B vaccine: ☐ NOT GIVEN ☐ GIVEN Nurse: _______________

If given: Date _____ Time _____ IM Site _____ Dose _____ Lot # _____

Hearing Screen Date: _____ OAE: L _____ R _____

PROGRESS NOTES

9000158 (10/05) NEWBORN ASSESSMENT (White - Chart Yellow ~ physician)

Figure 3. Standard Neonatal Assessment form.

THE COMPLETE PHYSICAL EXAMINATION

Examine a healthy newborn by anatomical region. It may be practical first to examine areas that require auscultation if the infant is quiet. As they may be somewhat irritable in early transition, undressing them or moving them around may be disruptive. In a seemingly healthy newborn most of the information is structural and may anticipate future problems. Figure 3 illustrates a standard newborn assessment hospital form. As many hospitals are going to electronic medical records, the health care professional will enter the requisite data into the specific template. Important future implications of an electronic health record lie in the ability to maintain and make information easily available to all care present and future providers for a newborn. This will result in better coordination of comprehensive care (2). The information on a physical examination of a newborn is available in many standard textbooks of pediatrics and neonatology (3,6).

Head

The average head circumference for a term newborn is approximately 34 cm. Observe the size and shape of the head. Transillumination should be available in a newborn nursery and is a helpful observation tool. Macrocephaly may be familial and benign, but may also be associated with Beckwith-Weidemann syndrome, Sotos Syndrome, neurocutaneous syndromes and chromosomal disorders such as fragile X or Klinefelter syndrome. Macrocephaly associated with enlarged bulging fontanelle should bring to mind obstruction to CSF flow often in posterior fossa abnormalities such as Dandy-Walker, Arnold Chiari and cystic malformations Are there areas that transilluminate, indicating abnormal collections of cerebrospinal fluid in the subdural, subarachnoid, intraventricular or posterior fossa regions? Microcephaly may be familial or genetic, but may also be associated with congenital infection (TORCH), maternal abuse of alcohol and cocaine, or intrauterine cerebrovascular accidents.

Are there any obvious malformations or protrusions such as an encephalocoele? Is the skull oddly shaped? Are there swellings and discolorations blisters and ulcerations possibly secondary to trauma of delivery or fetal monitoring? Palpate the head. Skull bones are mobile to the point of overriding each other while passing through the birth canal. There may also be skull molding (familiarly the "cone-head"). The initial head circumference may be small but will increase over the first few days as the molding and overriding resolve. Trauma of delivery may produce a cephalohematoma, actually a linear skull fracture, or a caput succedaneum, diffuse scalp edema which crosses a suture line. Check the sutures for premature closure, which will present as a sharp ridge along the suture line. This may not be apparent in the immediate newborn period. Occipital plagiocephaly occurs commonly today because of babies being placed in the "back to sleep" position, and may be asymmetric if the baby has torticollis or a strong tonic neck reflex. Compensatory frontal bossing on the ipsilateral side of the occipital flattening is benign. If not, it is important to consider premature closure of the coronal suture on the side of the plagiocephaly. Check the scalp for hair distribution. Are there any visible lesions or defects such as pits or areas of hair loss? Are there scalp abnormalities under the areas of hair loss (nevi, scars)? Note their location.

Eyes

The neonatal eye exam is chiefly observational, but can be difficult if the infant is agitated. Check general anatomy of the eye by assessing size, shape and position. Are they large (macrophthalmos), small (microphthalmos), slanted upwards or downwards, or too close (hypotelorism) or far apart (hypertelorism). If these findings are immediately obvious, it is important to check for other congenital anomalies and consider chromosomal disorders or other syndromic conditions. The most extreme form of hypotelorism is cyclopia with single midline facial structures and is invariably associated with midline brain abnormality (holoprosencephaly). Check the eyelids for edema and anatomic defects such as coloboma (cleft), ectropion (exposed palpebral conjunctivae). Eyelid edema is common in a healthy newborn and is usually associated with eye prophylaxis or dependent lymphatic flow from the recumbent position.

Obvious abnormalities of eyelashes or eyebrows, very long lashes, high-arched brows or single brow (synophrys) are associated with genetic abnormalities. The nasolacrimal duct system is frequently obstructed, (dacryostenosis), producing excess tearing. Drying tears may be yellow and crusty. Infection, dacryocystitis, has far more profuse exudates with a deeper yellow or more greenish hue. However, it is important to rule out other extrinsic causes such as cysts of the tear duct (dacryocystocoele), encephalocoeles, which may enter through the nasolacrimal system appearing as a mass in the inner canthal region, and hemangiomas.

Examine the sclerae, corneas and conjunctivae, irides and lenses. Are the sclerae white, or are they yellow (jaundice) or blue (osteogenesis imperfecta)? Often the pressure of delivery will produce scleral hemorrhages which form around the limbi and are benign and self-limiting. Corneal enlargement (>10mm in diameter) may be congenital glaucoma and merits immediate ophthalmologic referral, especially if associated with corneal opacity, tearing and photophobia. Refer corneal opacities due to cataracts or malformations (keratoconus, cornea plana) early so as to treat potential amblyopia. The conjunctivae may show redness or discharge from neonatal prophylaxis. Evaluate the irides and lenses with an ophthalmoscope. Although a good view of the ocular fundus in an awake newborn is virtually impossible, examination for red reflex (see figure 4) may demonstrate leukocoria (cat's eye, or white reflex) which carries a large differential diagnosis including retinoblastoma, cataracts, Coats' disease, persistent hyperplastic primary vitreous, retinal dysplasia and detachment, congenital infection and others, meriting immediate referral.

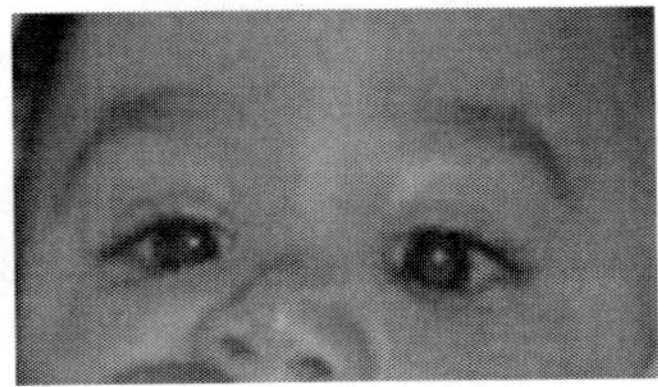

Figure 4. Normal red reflex.

The ophthalmoscope will reveal malformation of the iris such as aniridia (absence, often associated with hemihypertrophy and Wilm's tumor), pigmentary defects, colobomata, and Brushfield spots in Down syndrome. Most newborn irides are gray in color and the answer to the common question of "what color are my baby's eyes" should be to "wait until age 4 months when the color will be apparent." Dislocation of the lens may be associated with Marfan syndrome (superior) or homocystinuria (inferior). Normal newborns have vision, albeit highly myopic (20:400).

Many normal newborns will make eye contact or track and react to light by blinking or papillary response (miosis). Lack of these responses may raise suspicion of severe visual problems. Also, searching nystagmus may be a sign of cortical blindness in a newborn. A rotating drum with vertical lines on it will initiate the opticokinetic nystagmus useful to ascertain vision in a newborn. It is normal to have dysconjugate pupils at times up to age 6 months. However, it the pupils are always in an esotropic (toward the inner canthus) or exotropic (outer canthus) position, early referral is appropriate.

Ears

Inspect the morphology of the ears for size, shape and position. Is the external auditory meatus patent? Are there any abnormalities approximating the ear such as pre auricular pits or skin appendages? Otoscopy in the newborn is difficult because of the accumulation of vernix. Also, a small neonatal ear has a narrow S-shaped curve to the canal which is often difficult to negotiate. It is best to attempt this by placing and advancing the otoscope perpendicularly into the ear canal and pressing gently along the posterior aspect of the ear canal by moving the otoscope en bloc. Detecting tympanic membrane mobility is often difficult due to the softness of the ear canal which will move easily, creating the figure-ground illusion that the drum is moving. Most newborns undergo state-mandated auditory screening by otoacoustic emissions. Failure of this test should generate an immediate referral for further audiologic and otologic evaluation.

Enlarged ears (macrotia) or small ears (microtia) as an isolated finding may be hereditary or sporadic and are not significant. Enlarged ears should bring to mind chromosomal or syndromic conditions such as Fragile X syndrome, Cohen Syndrome and others. Small or atretic ears, similarly, may bespeak chromosomal or syndromic abnormalities such as Goldenhar, Treacher Collins, Trisomies 13, 18 and 21 among others. See the chapter on dysmorphology for more detail. Any atretic ear is deaf and early audiologic evaluation is necessary to prove otherwise.

Ears may be low set or malrotated. Draw an imaginary line that originates from the outer canthus, extending to the ear, originating from the slope of the ipsilateral eye. If the ear falls below that line, it is low-set. To assess rotation, the angle made by intersecting lines of the vertical axis of the head and the long axis of the pinna should be <20 degrees. Preauricular sinuses and pits unless associated with other anomalies are usually autosomally dominantly inherited traits and are benign. Many ears whose helices are over or under-folded, cup-ears are either positional due to uterine placement or sporadic and are of no clinical significance.

Nose

Inspect the nose for any malformations. As all newborns should have immediate suctioning at birth, failure of the catheter to pass through the nares may indicate choanal atresia. There may be congenital clefts or dimples. There may be deviation, often positional in nature. Excessively broad or narrow noses may be associated with chromosomal or syndromic conditions with other midline defects such as Crouzon, Treacher-Collins syndrome or holoprosencephaly. Nasal masses may be extrinsic and are associated with gliomas, encephalocoeles, dermoids and hemangiomas. Nasal obstruction can be a difficult problem for a newborn as they breathe through their noses and have difficulty adapting to mouth breathing. Other than genetic, syndromic and traumatic etiologies for nasal obstruction, consider inflammations and infection such as congenital syphilis, Chlamydia, rhinitis medicamentosa (maternal medication) and excessive amniotic fluid.

Mouth, tongue and throat

Check for any obvious malformations including the palate, gingivae and lips. Is there symmetry? Are there any clefts of the lip or palate? It is most important to palpate the palate for the possibility of a sub-mucous cleft. Mucosal cysts occur commonly on the palate (Epstein's pearls), the gingivae and buccal mucosa. Natal teeth may occur are often loose. Remove them to prevent aspiration. They may be the primary teeth, but sometimes are a third set. Is the philtrum well-formed? If too flat consider fetal alcohol syndrome especially if associated with cleft palate and IUGR. Does the mouth droop? If this occurs while crying, there could be absence of the depressor anguli oris muscle. If the mouth droops at all times with or without concomitant eyelid droop, consider cranial nerve palsies or obstetric injury. Check the tongue for size. Enlarged tongues should bring to mind hypothyroidism, Beckwith-Weidemann Syndrome or, rarely, storage diseases. The tongue may fall back (glossoptosis) causing airway obstruction, associated with retrognathia, indicative of Pierre-Robin syndrome. Look for ankyloglossia (tongue-tie), ranulas (salivary gland cysts below the tongue). Ankyloglossia, unless extreme (deep midline tongue furrow), usually does not require intervention; refer all ranulae for removal. Observe and auscultate carefully for any obstruction to respiration as a consequence of any of the above lesions.

Neck

Most newborn necks are quite short, but if abnormally so, or not mobile, may be a result of bony abnormalities as in Klippel-Feil syndrome. Check the neck for sinuses and tags in the post auricular region and along the anterior sternocleidomastoid border. A mass in the body of the sternocleidomastoid muscle indicates a possible bleed and may produce subsequent torticollis. Midline masses should bring to mind thyroid disorders such as thyroglossal duct cyst. Neck masses may compromise respiration and require immediate evaluation and may be dermoid cysts, hemangiomas, cystic hygromas, teratomas or reactive lymph nodes. Webbed necks should bring to mind Turner's syndrome, sometimes associated with generalized edema, or other collagen disorders that cause skin laxity such as Ehlers-Danlos syndrome. Observe and auscultate carefully to localize areas of upper airway compromise as a result of any of the above lesions.

Thorax

This area is conducive to inspection, palpation, percussion and auscultation.

Inspection: Look for any obvious malformations. Is the chest symmetrical? Is the diameter enlarged (air-trapping, intrathoracic masses, diaphragmatic hernia). Or is the diameter too narrow, (positional due to oligohydramnios, uterine positioning, skeletal dysplasia, absence of pectoralis muscle, Jeune's thoracodystrophy or muscle weakness such as spinal muscular atrophy). Is the baby breathing comfortably, at a normal rate (40-60 breaths per minute)? Normal term newborns will breathe, periodically, that is, slow or absent respirations for about 5 seconds, followed by rapid respirations. During pathologic breathing one may observe nasal flaring, chest retractions, head-bobbing or grunting. Note that suprasternal or sternal retractions indicate upper airway problems whereas intercostals and subcostal retractions indicate smaller airway problems. Asymmetric breathing patterns should bring to mind diaphragmatic or brachial palsy, pleural effusion, hemo-,chylo- or pnenuothorax. Are there any external dermatologic abnormalities such as nipples that are supernumerary, small or abnormally spaced? Think of Down syndrome (hypoplastic and narrow-spaced) or Turner Syndrome (shield-like chest, widely spaced). Look for skin color changes such as cyanosis or jaundice. As an adjunct to direct observation, transillumination may be helpful to evaluate the contents of the chest cavity (air, bowel, fluid).

Palpation: Palpate the clavicular areas for crepitus of fractures, or for ascent of air from a pneumomediastinum. Pain over the ribs indicates there may be a fracture. Palpation may demonstrate tactile fremitus as seen in pneumonia, or decreased fremitus in effusions. Feel the cardiac area for point of maximal intensity, hyperactive precordium or thrills. These may indicate significant congenital heart disease. Palpate breast tissue in the newborn. It is considered normal, secondary to maternal hormones and may accompany milk secretion (witch's milk). If there is erythema and tenderness, consider mastitis as a diagnosis.

Percussion: Small newborns make it difficult to localize by percussion.

Auscultation: Listen to the newborn with and without a stethoscope. The cry may be indicative. Is it lusty, weak, hoarse or high-pitched? Weak cries are non-specific and indicate many abnormalities (see section below on lethargy as a symptom in the newborn). Hoarse cries bespeak hypothyroidism and high-pitch cries should bring to mind neurological damage, kernicterus, or chromosomal abnormalities (especially Cri-du-chat syndrome). If the infant is tachypneic, is it noisy or quiet? Noisy tachypnea usually indicates upper airway involvement (rhonchi or stridor due to intrinsic or extrinsic tracheal compression) or lower airway involvement (grunting or wheezing), whereas quiet tachypnea usually has a CNS origin or can be from a respiratory compensation for a metabolic acidosis. Cardiac failure in the newborn may present with tachypnea and grunting or wheezing, along with sweating and easy fatiguability.

The stethoscope is an important tool for diagnosing cardiac or respiratory problems. Listen for sounds that may confirm what we hear without the stethoscope such as rhonchi. The stethoscope may help localize the sounds to the pharynx, trachea or bronchi. Listen for rales and wheezing. Listen for heart tones, their intensity, rhythm and the different components of the first and second cardiac sounds and adventitial sounds such as murmurs, rubs or gallops. This may be quite difficult in an infant whose heart rate averages about 140 beats per minute. Keep in mind that a newborn with severe congenital heart disease may demonstrate no cardiac murmur until there are differential pressures developed between the left and right side of the heart during the first several days of life.

Abdomen

Inspection: The newborn abdomen is proportionally larger and rounder than that of an adult. Furthermore, as the baby swallows air and food after birth, the abdominal girth increases. Does the abdomen appear distended? If so, does it originate from high or low intestinal obstruction, Hirschsprung's disease (aganglionic megacolon) or extra-intestinal pathology such as meconium peritonitis, ascites, hemoperitoneum or pneumoperitoneum? Observe the abdominal skin for discoloration such as jaundice or cyanosis (central). Venous markings are normal on a newborn abdomen, but should not be tortuous or distended. Check the umbilical area for hernias. Large hernias may indicate hypothyroidism. Very large umbilical protrusions may be omphalocoeles necessitating immediate repair. Abdominal contents may protrude through the abdominal, more often to the right of the umbilicus in gastroschisis, also requiring immediate attention. Count the umbilical vessels, which should consist of one vein and two arteries. If there is only one artery, is it an isolated finding, or are there other congenital anomalies present? If there is leakage from the umbilicus, think of urine through a patent urachus or stool through a patent omphalomesenteric duct. Separation of the rectus abdominus muscles with some bulging is normal for a newborn (diastasis recti). A flat (scaphoid) abdomen should bring to mind diaphragmatic hernia. Loose floppy abdominal skin may indicate underdevelopment of the abdominal wall as in the Eagle-Barrett (prune-belly) syndrome also associated with genital abnormalities.

Palpation: Check for abdominal masses. The most common cause for a palpable abdominal mass in a newborn is cystic dysplasia of the kidney. Other renal causes include: polycystic kidneys (autosomal recessive or dominant), uretero-pelvic obstruction, renal vein thrombosis, Wilms' tumor, bladder obstruction, or neurogenic bladder. Adrenal causes include hemorrhage, neuroblastoma and others. Gastrointestinal causes are duplications, cysts and lymphangiomas. Liver enlargement may be caused by hematomas, tumors (benign or malignant) or metastatic disease, especially from neuroblastoma. Biliary causes for abdominal masses include choledochal cysts and hydrops of the gallbladder. Genital tract problems include ovarian cyst or tumor and hydrometrocolpos, usually from an imperforate hymen.

Percussion: Although it is difficult to localize pathology by this technique, it is helpful to outline organ margins and to determine if there is excess air, either extra or intra-intestinal.

Auscultation: Newborns often have less active bowel sounds until feeding is well-established. However, overactive bowel sounds may be indicative of an intestinal obstruction and absent bowel sounds for several minutes may indicate peritonitis.

The perineum

Female genitalia: A normal female newborn may demonstrate edema of the labia, especially with a breech-presentation, and this resolves spontaneously. A creamy vaginal discharge, sometimes streaked with blood is due to maternal hormones and is also within normal limits. Hymenal anatomy has many normal variants including clefts, cysts, crescents and ridges. However an imperforate hymen (bluish bulge) causes hemato-metrocolpos and requires immediate attention. Also, a septate hymen may indicate duplications higher in the genital tract. Virilized female genitalia present with clitoromegaly and labial fusion. Causes for this include fetal: congenital adrenal hyperplasia, virilizing tumors of the ovary or adrenal glands, maternal: tumors with hormone production affecting the fetus, exogenous: progestogens, stilbestrol and androgens. Consult the endocrinology chapter for further discussion.

Male genitalia: The normal penis should be >2.5 cm. Often it is buried in a preputial fat pad and appears deceptively small. Pressure on the mons pubis region with penile stretching will usually reveal a normal penile length. A true micropenis should bring to mind hypopituitarism, often accompanied by hypoglycemia. Hypoadrenalism and other genetic syndromes may also cause micropenis. Make certain the penile opening is located close to the tip. Sometimes it is located ventrally, often associated with incomplete foreskin and chordee (ventral shortening) and requires surgical repair. In more severe forms of hypospadias the meatus is located on the penile shaft, the peno-scrotal junction or the scrotum. These require immediate attention. Epispadias is the insufficient closure of the dorsal aspect of the penis and is sometimes associated with exstrophy of the bladder. Check the scrotum for size and contour. Bifid scrotum, hooded scrotum may be a normal variant if not associated with other anomalies. An enlarged scrotum may be due to normal edema after delivery (especially breech) and resolves spontaneously. Hydrocoele is the most common cause of an enlarged scrotum, is not associated with discomfort and transilluminates easily. Neonatal hernias may appear as a hydrocoele, but do not transilluminate. These should be referred for repair, whereas most hydrocoeles will resolve with no intervention.

Infections and torsions are associated with discomfort and require immediate attention. Tumors are rare in newborns. Make certain the testes are palpable bilaterally and are descended. Normal testicular volume for a newborn is >1.1 ml. Testes may be high in the scrotum or inguinal canal and one must follow them for eventual descent. If the testes are non-palpable and if there are any other genital abnormalities consider congenital adrenal hyperplasia (3ß-hydroxyseroid dehydrogenase deficiency), hermaphroditism, androgen deficiency or resistance or syndromic conditions. Consult the endocrine chapter for further detail.

Ambiguous genitalia: Sometimes it is difficult to determine the gender of a newborn immediately at birth. Consult the endocrine chapter for further discussion.

The back

Inspect the back for obvious masses or deformities. Spina bifida may present either covered with skin or open. Other causes for midline masses include sacrococcygeal teratomas and lipomas. Check the entire posterior midline for dimples or sinuses. If they occur further than 2 cm away from the anus they may well communicate with the central nervous system and refer them immediately. Abnormal tufts of hair in the sacral region may bespeak spina bifida, tethered cord or other CNS abnormalities. Pilonidal sinuses and cysts occur within 2 cm of the anus and are benign if the examiner sees the floor of the dimple. If not, ultrasound is necessary to delineate the anatomy. Check the anus for patency. 99% of normal newborns should pass meconium within the first 48 hours of life. Congenital scoliosis is not normal and it is necessary to image the spine for abnormalities.

Extremities

Upper extremities: Check the arms, hands and fingers for obvious deformities such as hypoplasia, amputation phocomelia. Are there fractures? This may indicate osteogenesis imperfecta. Are the extremities stiff and malformed as in arthrogryposis? Count fingers. Isolated syndactyly or polydactyly especially with an extra fifth finger located proximally is usually a benign autosomally dominant condition. However, polydactyly may be associated with many other genetic and syndromic conditions especially when originating from the thumb.

Check where the fingers are set, especially the thumb. Consult the chapter on genetics for further detail. Are there any signs of brachial palsy, Erb's with weakness of shoulder abduction and external rotation and weakness of elbow flexion and wrist extension (porter's tip syndrome), or Klumpke's with clawing of involved hand (see figures 5 and 6).

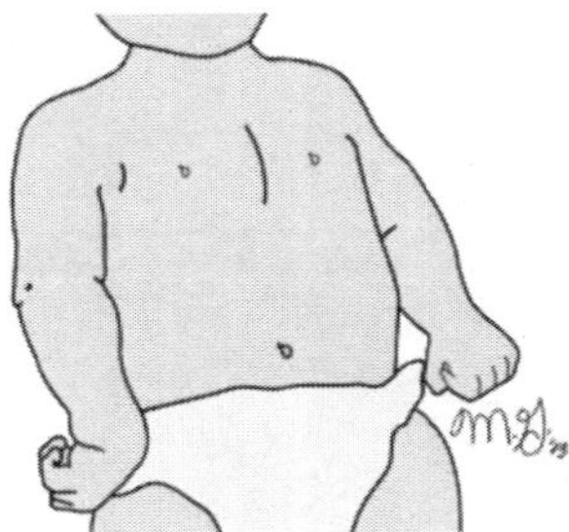

Figure 5. Erb's palsy.

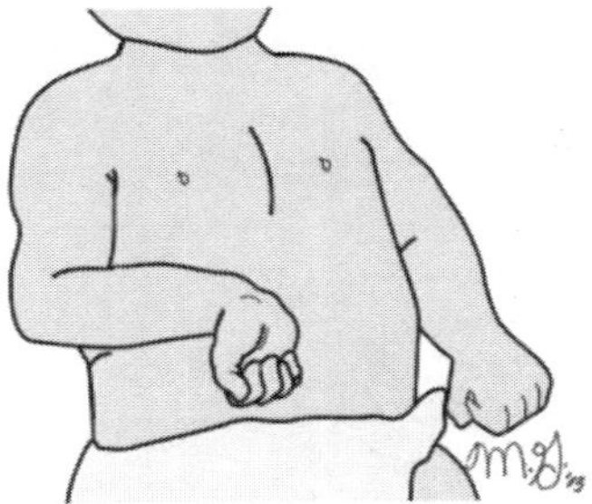

Figure 6. Klumpke's palsy.

Lower extremities: Inspect the legs for obvious deformities as with the upper extremity examination. An extreme form of lower limb dysplasia may be a consequence of the caudal regression syndrome seen in infants of diabetic mothers. Evaluate the lower extremity from the hips down to the toes. Developmental dysplasia of the hip may appear in more severe cases as a shortened, medially rotated leg with asymmetric gluteal folds and a +Galeazzi sign with unequal knee height (see figure 7). Always perform a Barlow (with hips adducted, grab femur encircling the knee and push posteriorly) and follow with the Ortolani maneuver (abduct the hips). The Barlow maneuver, pushing the femur down toward the exam table, will force the hip out of the socket and the Ortolani maneuver, abduction of the hips, will relocate it with a "klunk" sensation (see figures 8 and 9). Internally or externally rotated femora, internal tibial torsion or in-curved feet (metatarsus adductus) may be normal in newborns as a result of fetal positioning, especially if the limbs are flexible and easily manipulated into a normal position. If the foot is permanently in the equinovarus position (forefoot supination, varus angulation and medially-facing soles), this is a club-foot to refer immediately for casting. With any extremity malformation, always check for any spinal abnormality that may be a cause.

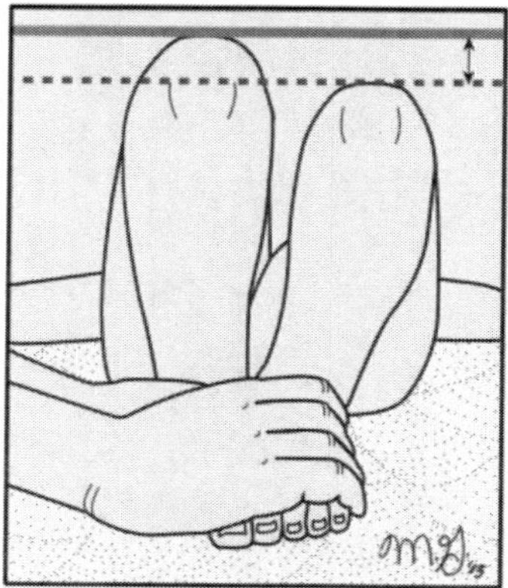

Figure 7. Galeazzi sign.

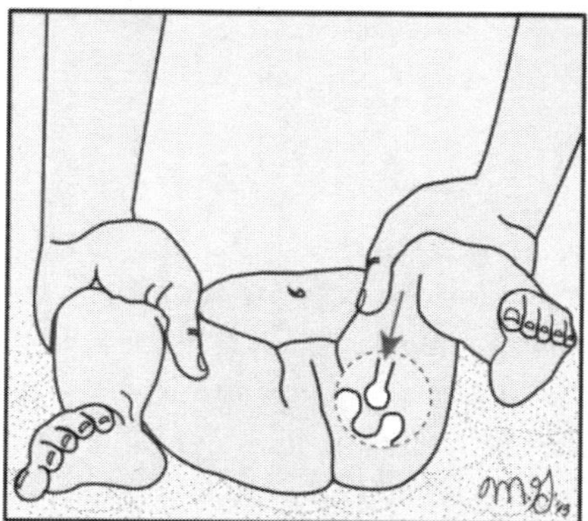

Figure 8. Barlow maneuver.

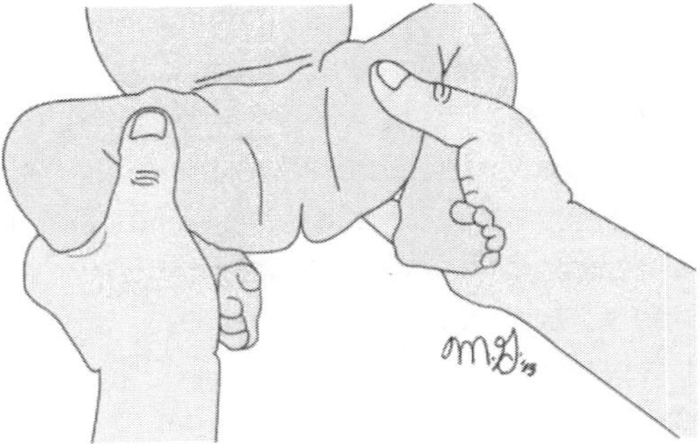

Figure 9. Ortolani Maneuver.

NEUROLOGICAL EXAM

A term newborn exam must take into consideration cerebral, cranial nerve, sensory and motor functioning. We will present a basic neurologic evaluation and please refer to the chapter on neurology for further detail.

Cerebral: Although they cannot answer our questions, they demonstrate varying levels of consciousness and alertness. Objective scales assess newborn states, ranging from coma to fully awakened state. Soon after birth some newborns may show preference for their mothers or other familiar faces by making more prolonged and intense eye contact. Some may orient toward sound. Is the baby alert or sleepy, active or lethargic, tense or relaxed, quiet, fussy or tremulous? Are there any abnormal movements such as athetosis (writhing)? If the baby is fussy is he/she consolable? Does he/she seem to respond to cuddling at any time? Remember that a normal newborn's state of alertness will fluctuate, so it may be necessary to do prolonged or several evaluations. Some newborns are capable of making seemingly purposeful defensive maneuvers. For example, they will be able to bat at a cloth if put over their faces. Some will extend their necks while being held for assessment of a retinal light reflex, thus making it even more difficult for the examiner.

Sensory: Newborns see, albeit myopically, and hear. Many newborns can make eye-contact and can follow around the midline, the presence of which may be reassuring to the examiner. Newborn hearing screening measuring oto-acoustic emissions is routine in every state. Immediate follow up of an abnormal screen is important. Newborns definitely feel pain and discomfort and will withdraw reflexively and cry. Thus, proper anesthesia or analgesia is mandatory for all procedures.

Motor: As in any neurological examination, evaluate general tone (normal, hypotonic, hypertonic) (see figure 2) and posture (normal, opisthotonic, decorticate, decerebrate). Newborns generally maintain a mildly flexed position of all four extremities. Posture may be asymmetric with preference to one side, but tone should be normal. Look carefully for any evidence of focal weakness, unilateral or bilateral.

Reflexes: Newborns are more reflexive than at any other stage of their lives. It is not entirely clear why newborns have them, but there are some anthropologic explanations such as primitive survival or instinctive preparation for fright/flight. Newborn reflexes are helpful for assessing spinal function, both sensory and motor, but may be present and normal in newborns with anencephaly, and thus, are not helpful for assessing cerebral damage. There have been more than eighty newborn reflexes described. We will illustrate some of the more commonly-used ones often described as active reflexes. Abnormalities usually present with overreaction, under-reaction or asymmetry.

Suck: The baby will suck automatically if a finger or pacifier is placed on the roof of his/her mouth.

Rooting: When the examiner strokes the cheek or corner of the mouth the baby will turn his/her head toward the source and attempts to suck.

Moro: After gently lifting the baby by the arms with the head still on the mattress, release your grip so the baby's back falls to the underlying surface. The baby will have a double response – first arm abduction and elbow extension, then arm adduction, elbow flexion and finger curling (see figure 10).

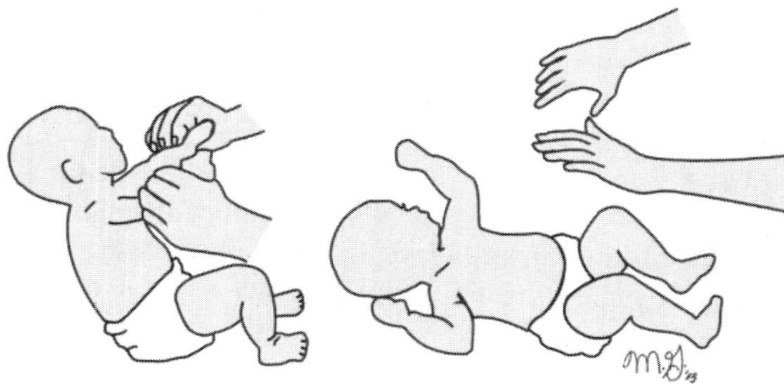

Figure 10. Moro response.

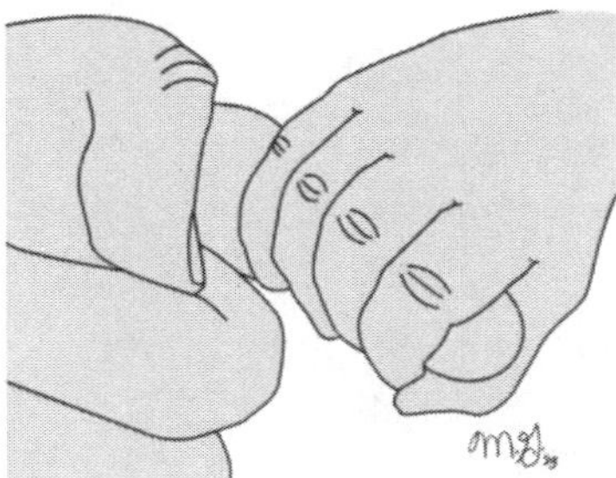

Figure 11. Palmar grasp response.

Startle: Often confused with the Moro reflex, elicit it similarly, but the baby will flex the arms only and have a generalized startle. Repetition will habituate this response.

Palmer or plantar grasp: The baby will automatically flex the fingers or toes onto anything placed in his/her palm or sole (see figures 11and 12).

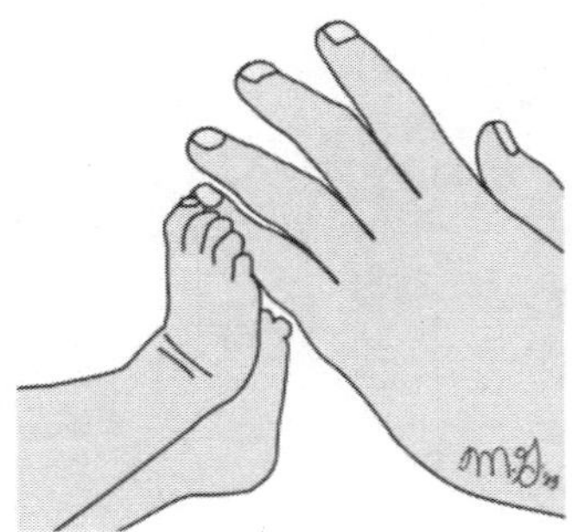

Figure 12. Plantar grasp response.

Tonic neck: When the infant is relaxed turn the head to one side. The infant will assume the "en garde" position with the arm that would hold the sword on the same side the head faces, while the other arm is flexed and held up straight alongside the head (see figure 13).

Traction: Place fingers in the infant's palms. As he/she grasps, lifting the baby will elicit elbow and neck flexion. Similarly, pulling the infant to a sitting position or raising the infant from the supine position from the shoulders will also elicit neck flexion (see figure 14).

                     Arthur N Feinberg

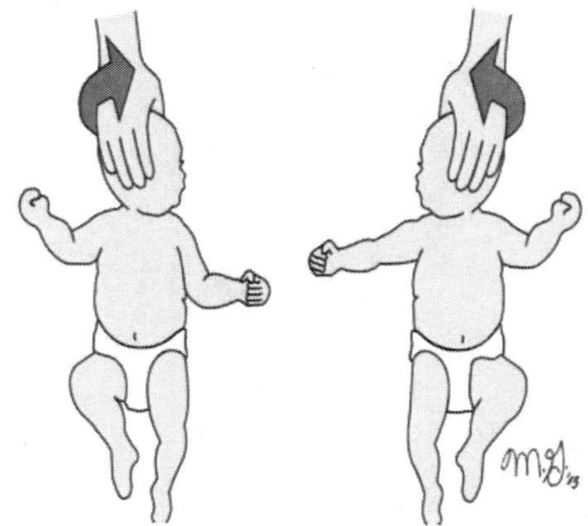

Figure 13. Tonic neck reflex.

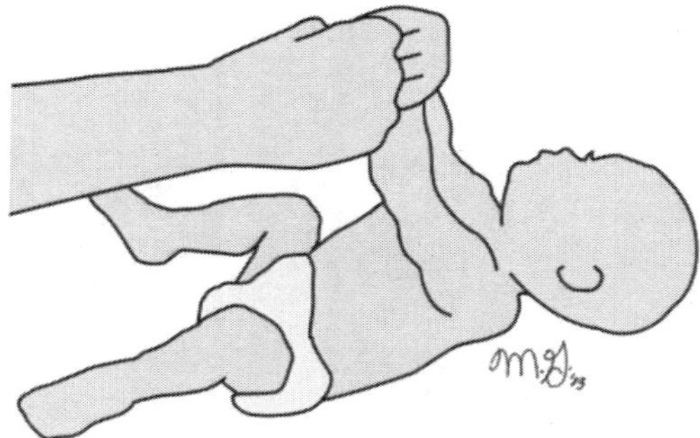

Figure 14. Traction reflex.

Perez response: Hold the infant in the prone position grasping under the abdomen Gentle rubbing up the spine will elicit flexion of the extremities and extension of the neck. Similarly, elicit the Vollmer by rubbing down the spine and will cause flexion of the lower extremities and extension of the back.

Galant response: Hold infant in prone position as in the Perez response and rub lightly along the flank. The baby will move his/her buttocks toward the ipsilateral side. This reflex is particularly amusing to older siblings (see figure 15).

Magnet response: Grasp both heels and press thumbs on balls of infant's feet thus dorsiflexing them. The baby will extend the legs.

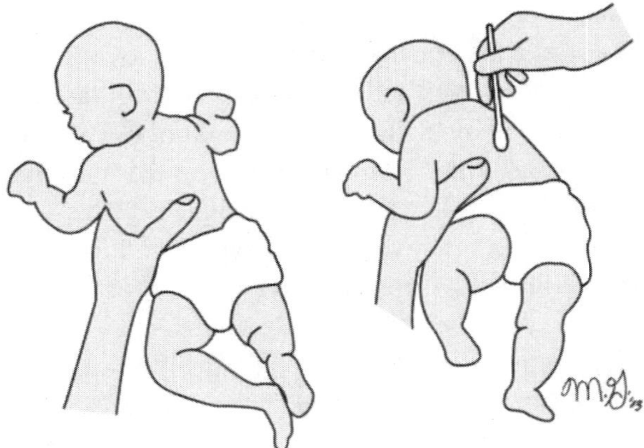

Figure 15. Galant response.

Placing response: Hold the infant upright with both hands around the thorax and then gently place both feet on the surface. He/she will attempt to extend both legs and straighten the trunk(see figure 16).

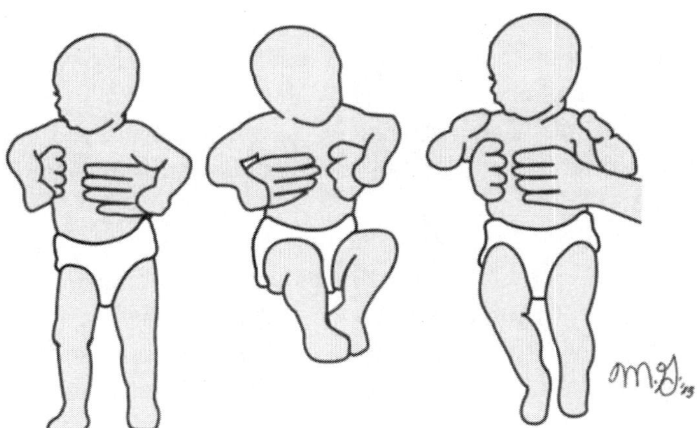

Figure 16. Placing response.

Stepping: Hold infant upright with both feet on the surface of the table. Move infant from side to side to elicit stepping movements. Also have the infant rub the dorsum of the foot under the edge of a bassinet or a table top. The infant will bring his/her foot up on the surface in a walking-like manner. This is the second best reflex for an older sibling's amusement.

Crossed extension reflex: With the baby lying supine, straighten out one leg at the knee and stroke the plantar surface of that foot with your other hand. The opposite leg should first flex and abduct, the toes will fan and then the leg will extend and adduct, moving its foot toward the foot that was stroked.

Babinski reflex: Scratching the lateral aspect of the foot will elicit dorsiflexion of the big toe and fanning of all the others.

Ankle clonus: Abruptly press your thumb on the ball of a foot to produce sudden dorsiflexion. Normally, there should be <5 beats of clonus.

Also note there are many tests for muscle tone that are passive. Examples are scarf sign, heel-to ear maneuver, popliteal angle and wrist-window. They also assess tone in gestational age assessment (see figure 1). In summary note that the material provided in this section is considered traditional and is also available in many standard textbooks and articles (1-3,6).

MONITORING THE NORMAL NEWBORN

Normal growth patterns: Because a newborn is comprised of 80% water, all normal newborns may lose up to 10% of birth weight during hospitalization. It is important to follow up newborns to assure they reach birth weight by no later than 2 weeks of age. Then they should be gaining 20-30g/day. Also note many newborns will have a seemingly large increase in head circumference from birth to discharge due to overriding sutures resuming a normal conformation.

Vital signs: During transition, the newborn respiratory and pulse rate can be quite variable. Early tachypnea can be considered normal as the newborn rids his/her lungs of excess fluid. The newborn heart rate eventually stabilizes to an average of 140-160 beats per minute (bpm), but may go to as low as 90 bpm during sleep. Respiratory rates eventually stabilizes after transition to an average of 40-60/min. Normal core temperature is 36.5-37.5°C7 It is always important to evaluate the color of an infant. Recently, more institutions are going to routine screening for cyanosis by pulse oximetry and at present seven states have mandated this.

Feeding patterns: A normal newborn will require few calories in the first three days of life as their metabolic rate is slow (approximately 60 kcal/kg). However, note a marked subsequent increase in metabolic rate such that caloric needs reach a maximum at age one week (up to 140 kcal/kg). A normal healthy newborn will increase intake to meet these needs, especially, if nursing, as mother's milk usually comes at age 3 days. Please refer to the chapter on nutrition and breastfeeding.

Voiding and stooling: Newborns typically start with black (actually very dark green) very sticky meconium, progresses to "transitional" stools at about 2-3 days (mushy green-brown) and then on to typical newborn stool that look like mustard seeds in water. A newborn should pass stools by 48 hours; otherwise there should be concerns for intestinal obstruction or Hirschsprung's disease. Similarly, a newborn should pass urine by 24 hours of life; otherwise genitourinary problems must be entertained. It is important to be sure a newborn is passing urine and stool, as often they can mix with each other and be difficult to detect. Infants may pass orange or brick-colored urine which represents uric acid crystals which should not be misconstrued for blood (2).

Jaundice: All newborns receive a screening bilirubin test during the first 24 hours of life. The standard nomogram is quite predictive of who will be at risk for significantly elevated levels of bilirubin (see figure 17). Note that the risk zone the patient falls in at the time of the test, in hours of age, represents the risk (low intermediate, high) of serum bilirubin level increasing to the 95 percentile eventually. Please consult the section below on jaundice for further detail (8).

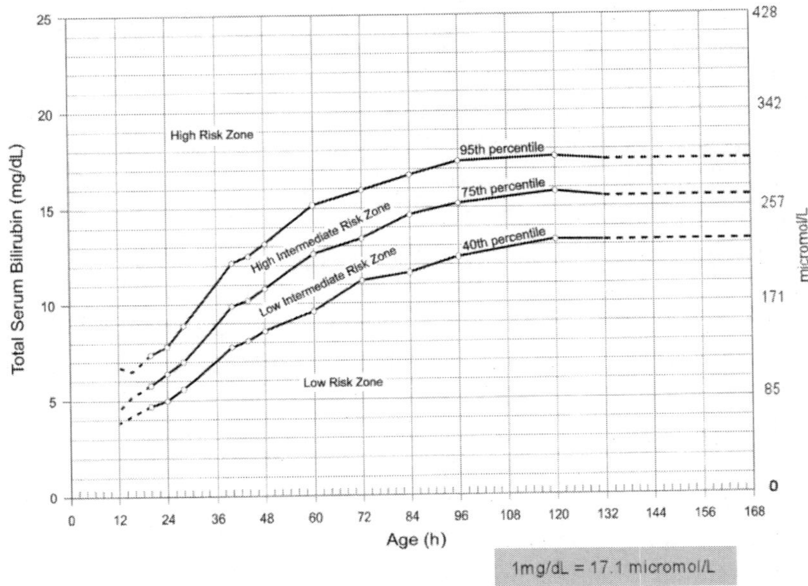

Figure 17. Bilirubin nomogram.

Temperament: Newborns will often show patterns regarding reactivity, rhythmicity, approach-withdrawal, adaptability, attention, intensity, distractibility, mood threshold of response and ability to self-regulate. Research has demonstrated a persistence of these patterns throughout life. Although there is a vast spectrum of these characteristics, none of them is defined as inherently pathologic. More important than merely describing characteristics is to determine how parents react to these traits and to guide them into matching temperaments in order to create the best possible "fit." More on this appears in the chapter on anticipatory guidance and in the psychosocial issues section (9).

COMMON PROBLEMS IN A TERM NEWBORN

Growth problems

Small for gestational age: Small for gestational age is defined as >2 standard deviations below the mean. In full term newborns this is 2500 grams or less. Maternal, fetal or placental problems may contribute toward this Obtain a maternal history, asking for hypoxia (cardiac or pulmonary disease), hypertension, sickle cell anemia, advanced diabetes mellitus, malnutrition and drug abuse including tobacco. Gross and microscopic examination of the placenta will be helpful to assess for scarring, infarction, infection, tumor or insufficient size or surface area. Newborn causes are chromosomal or syndromic disorders, multiple gestation congenital infection (TORCH) and insulin deficiency.

Large for gestational age: Large for gestational age is defined as >2 standard deviations above the mean, or 4,000 gm in a term newborn. Is the mother diabetic? Infants of diabetic mothers are long and "jowly" appearing due to the action of their own excess production of insulin as a response to maternal hyperglycemia. Check for many other anatomic problems associated with infants of diabetic mothers such as polyhydramnios, microcolon (abdominal distention), congenital heart disease (asymmetric septal hypertrophy, cono-truncal anomalies) and caudal regression syndrome. Syndromic causes of large for gestational age babies include Beckwith-Weidemann (omphalocoele, large tongue, organomegaly) and Soto syndrome (cerebral gigantism, associated with large head circumference in a newborn).

Temperature instability

Newborns, especially small ones have difficulty maintaining their temperature due to lack of fat and immaturity of the hypothalamic thermostat.

Hyperthermia: Any report from a neonatal nurse regarding fever in a newborn merits immediate attention. The febrile newborn is septic unless proven otherwise and the physician should have a low threshold for pursuing an evaluation. Always review prenatal history especially maternal carriage of group B streptococcus and appropriateness of antibiotic prophylaxis. Most nurseries have protocols for immediate newborn evaluation for all mothers who are colonized. Neonatal sepsis is protean in manifestation and may appear as hypothermia, lethargy, poor feeding, vomiting abdominal distention and jaundice. If clinical suspicion for sepsis is high, a full evaluation should be conducted including CBC, urinalysis, chest x-ray and cultures of blood, cerebrospinal fluid and urine. CRP (C reactive protein) is a non-specific test of inflammation and should not be used in the initial evaluation, although levels over 4mg% may militate toward the diagnosis. There are non-pathologic causes for hyperthermia including over-wrapping and maternal epidural anesthesia, but do not attribute fever to these alone unless the newborn is otherwise asymptomatic and free of risk criteria for sepsis. Keep in mind that sepsis is not relegated to bacteria and it is important to consider viral infections, especially Enteerovirus and Herpes hominis.

Hypothermia: Hypothermia may result from inadequate swaddling, but also, in conjunction with other symptoms as mentioned above under hyperthermia may also indicate sepsis, and may be a more ominous sign than hyperthermia. Lower neonatal reserves of glycogen and fat often result in hypoglycemia but consider inborn errors of metabolism when it is associated with vomiting and lethargy.

Tachypnea

General overview: Neonatal tachypnea has many anatomic origins, including respiratory, cardiac, and neurological. There also may be many origins including infectious and metabolic. When confronted with a tachypneic newborn, always ask further questions as to the time of onset (birth, or later). Is the tachypnea deep or shallow? Is it symmetric? Is the patient comfortable, or not? Check the progression (static, worsening) and degree of distress (grunting, flaring or retracting). Is there accompanying cyanosis or pallor? Is the newborn alert and vigorous, irritable or lethargic? Is there fever or vomiting? Is there a peculiar odor to the baby?

Always review the prenatal and delivery history for any clue pointing to infection, or trauma. Examine the newborn carefully for any signs of upper airway obstruction (stridor), absence or asymmetry of breath sounds, rhonchi, rales or wheezes. Do a complete cardiac examination, listening for heart rate, murmurs, intensity of heart tones and peripheral pulses.

It is important to prioritize the evaluation of the tachypneic newborn depending on the suspected diagnosis and severity of the illness. Pursue pulmonary, cardiac or neurological causes if the history and physical exam lead to it. Vomiting, lethargy, irritability and temperature instability are non-specific and should prompt evaluation for infectious, metabolic or neurological etiologies. We outline diagnostic considerations below:

Respiratory: Is there evidence of upper airway blockage? Consider choanal atresia, nasal trauma or any congenital malformation or compression of the tracheo-bronchial tree (stenosis, or aberrant vessels or aortic arch remnants compressing the area). Always have a low threshold for ordering a chest x-ray on a tachypneic newborn. It is rapid, economical and provides much valuable information. Consider aspiration syndromes (vernix, stomach contents, meconium), pneumonia, extra-pulmonary accumulation of air (pneumothorax), blood (hemothorax) or lymph (chylothorax). Congenital abnormalities of lung formation may include emphysema and cystic adenomatoid malformation. If a newborn remains cyanotic in spite of O2 administration, think of persistent fetal circulation (pulmonary hypertension). This is known as the hyperoxia test. Hyaline membrane disease is very rare in a term newborn, but may be associated with polyhydramnios, caesarean section delivery and has a higher incidence in infants of diabetic mothers.

More commonly a newborn will be tachypneic due to slow evacuation of lung fluid. The symptoms occur immediately after birth. There may be flaring and retracting, but the infants do not appear very ill. This is transient tachypnea of the newborn and is benign and self-limiting.

Cardiac: It is important to note that absence of a heart murmur in a tachypneic newborn does not eliminate the possibility of severe cardiac disease. Many murmurs depend upon a differential pressure between the left and right circuits, which has not developed as yet. If cyanosis is present perform a hyperoxia test, and if the newborn is unable to improve the O_2 saturation, cyanotic heart disease is a definite possibility. It is important to pursue a cardiac evaluation in a timely fashion and to administer prostaglandins to maintain patency of the ductus arteriosus pending definitive treatment. The most common cyanotic lesions are the "five T's," Transposition, Tetralogy of Fallot (less likely in the immediate newborn period), Tricuspid atresia, Truncus arteriosus and Total anomalous pulmonary venous return. Other lesions such as pulmonary atresia may also cause cyanosis. Another significant ductal dependent lesion is hypoplastic left heart syndrome which also requires prostaglandins and rapid diagnosis. All newborns with cyanotic heart disease merit immediate evaluation by a pediatric cardiologist.

Cardiac failure is very rare in the term newborn nursery, and is most commonly due to critical aortic stenosis. It will manifest as lethargy, poor feeding, pallor and diaphoresis. If a newborn has an apparent chromosomal syndrome, always look carefully for congenital heart disease. This is especially true for newborns with Down syndrome. Evaluate them immediately for endocardial cushion (av communis) defect regardless of any physical findings. Consult the chapter on cardiology for more detail.

Neurological: Tachypnea of neurological origin is notably quiet. Sometimes the normal stress of delivery will cause a temporary metabolic acidosis for which the newborn compensates by tachypnea. This is benign and self-limiting. However, serious neurological injury, e.g., intracranial hemorrhage, will often present as tachypnea, lethargy, or irritability. Similarly, neonatal meningitis presents as such and must be diagnosed and treated immediately.

Infectious: Tachypnea may be less than specific than hyperthermia, especially if isolated. Raise suspicion for sepsis if there are predisposing risk factors or if the infant appears even slightly ill. If clinical suspicion is relatively low, some experts suggest a "modified" sepsis workup, leaving out a lumbar puncture because of the low risk for meningitis in a newborn that is not strongly symptomatic. Others suggest a full evaluation because of differences in management between sepsis and meningitis. As with hyperthermia, do not forget to include viruses, especially Herpes.

Metabolic: Tachypnea may be a non-specific indicator of general stress and may be secondary to hypoglycemia, abnormal electrolytes including Calcium and Magnesium. Always consider inborn errors of metabolism especially in newborns that are lethargic or vomiting or have a distinct odor to them. In these instances tachypnea is a respiratory compensation for severe metabolic acidosis. Consult the chapter on neurology for an approach to these patients. Review the cardiology and pulmonology chapters for further elaboration.

Apnea

Apnea in a term healthy newborn is relatively rare. It is defined as a period of >20sec and should not be confused with normal periodic breathing due to relative immaturity of CO2 receptor centers in the medulla. Consider respiratory causes as outlined under "tachypnea", hypoxia and neurological causes such as seizures, intracranial hemorrhage, herniation, infarction, neuromuscular disease, phrenic nerve paralysis, toxins and medications. Infectious causes include sepsis of all etiologies. Metabolic causes as discussed above as well as hypothermia are considerations.

Cyanosis

Cyanosis in the newborn is usually cardiac or respiratory in origin. See previous discussions for respiratory and cardiac causes of tachypnea as well as the pulmonary and cardiac chapters of this book. Polycythemia, methemoglobinemia will appear as cyanosis and are often mistaken for cardio-pulmonary conditions. Cyanosis may be factitious (acrocyanosis, with concomitant falsely low pulse-oximetry readings due to poor circulation).

Heart murmurs

As discussed above, absence of a heart murmur does not rule out severe congenital heart disease. Soft upper sternal border murmurs are frequently due to a patent ductus arteriosus, which is benign and self-limiting. Administration of oxygen (hyperoxia test) will cause the murmur to disappear due to spasm of the ductus in response to O_2. If a newborn is symptomatic (tachypnea, cyanosis), heart murmurs merit immediate attention with pediatric cardiac consultation. Observe an asymptomatic newborn with a heart murmur, evaluate and refer as needed. See the chapter on cardiology for more details.

Poor feeding, vomiting and constipation

Poor feeding/lethargy: This is usually a non-specific finding and may have multiple causes including infectious, metabolic cardiac and neurological as discussed above. Pathology of the GI tract is relatively rare as a cause.

Vomiting: This occurs frequently in a newborn and it is important to assess the nature in order to develop a sensible diagnostic plan. On what day of life did it start? Does it occur immediately after feeding? Is it projectile? Is there any blood, bile or stool? Is the baby ill-appearing? We outline causes of vomiting below:

Upper gastrointestinal: It is best to break down gastrointestinal etiologies of vomiting into upper and lower causes. If vomiting occurs right after feeding, consider the upper GI tract. A common cause is Tracheo-esophageal fistula, the most common type of which is a blind esophageal pouch where immediately at birth a suction catheter will not pass. Consider GER, motility disorders as achalasia and hiatal hernia. Gastric causes of vomiting include congenital abnormalities such as pyloric atresia, volvulus, duplication and antral webs. These are often suspected because of abdominal distention associated with polyhydramnios and an excessive amount of amniotic fluid suctioned from the stomach at birth. Hypertrophic pyloric stenosis is very rare in the term newborn nursery, but may occur in the neonatal period especially with a history of macrolide administration. Duodenal atresia is a significant cause of vomiting in the newborn, and like the above gastric causes will present with abdominal distention as well. Other causes of duodenal obstruction include annular pancreas and Ladd's bands. Bilious vomiting may be due to obstruction at or below the sphincter of Oddi and merits immediate investigation.

Mid gastrointestinal: Think of ileal or jejunal atresias as well as Ladd's bands, malrotation, volvulus and intestinal duplications. Intussusception occurs very rarely in the immediate newborn period.

Lower gastrointestinal: Vomiting may not occur until day 3 of life and may be feculent in nature. Absence of stool or constipation often occurs. 99% of normal term newborn should pass stool within 48 hours. Stooling patterns are variable ranging from once every other day to 8 times/day. Consistency is also variable with breast fed babies having mushier stools. Always perform at least a visual examination of the anus for patency. Colonic obstruction may be due to stenosis, atresia, duplications or external from Ladd bands, malrotation and volvulus. Aganglionic megacolon (Hirschsprung's disease) and meconium ileus (cystic fibrosis) are always considerations. Sometimes newborns appear obstructed from a hard meconium plug which, when removed by enema administration of gastrografin will produce immediate relief. This condition is not associated with cystic fibrosis. Consult the chapter on neonatal gastroenterology for further information.

Non-gastrointestinal: Keep in mind vomiting can be non-specific and is associated with infectious, neurological or metabolic disorders as discussed above. Constipation can have metabolic causes such as hypothyroidism.

Irritability/jitteriness

Irritability or jitteriness in the newborn may be normal in a small thin baby. Often trauma of a normal delivery may leave a newborn slightly irritable as they make the adjustment to extra-uterine life. More severe or protracted symptoms should bring to mind metabolic/toxic (hypoglycemia hypo/hypernatremia, hypocalcemia, drug-withdrawal) or neurological disorders (congenital malformation, trauma, infection). Consider causes of hypoglycemia such as hyperinsulinism (infant of diabetic mother, nesidioblastosis, Beckwith-Weidemann syndrome), depleted glycogen stores, endocrine (hyperinsulinism, hypopituituarism, hypoadrenalism), and metabolic disorders (gluconeogenesis, fatty acid breakdown). Neonatal seizures (see below) are often subtle in nature and may appear as hyper-irritability. Severely jaundiced newborns may manifest kernicterus as irritability, high-pitch cry, deafness, sunset eyes and chorioathetosis. Hypocalcemia may be secondary to low birth weight, phosphate overload hypoparathyroidism (consider Di George syndrome) or renal failure. Consult the neurology, renal and endocrine chapters for more detail.

Seizures

Neonatal seizures, as in older children may be tonic, clonic or myoclonic, but also may be subtle in presentation and appear as irritability, stereotyped movements such as lip-smacking, blinking or bicycling. Because of deficiency of myelination in the newborn, symptoms and EEG changes may be quite variable. The most common cause of neonatal seizures is hypoxic-ischemic encephalopathy. Consider congenital malformations, CNS trauma (intracranial hemorrhage), infection (sepsis, meningitis, viral infection such as TORCH) and metabolic conditions such those discussed above under irritability/jitteriness as well as inborn errors of metabolism (see neurology chapter for further detail). Of particular interest in the neonatal period is pyridoxine deficiency which will respond dramatically to its administration. After ruling out the above causes, neonatal seizures may be benign as in familial seizures (autosomal dominant and self-limited to about 6 months) and "fifth-day fits" which last for about one day and are without sequelae. The chapter on neonatal neurology contains further information.

Pallor or plethora

Newborns are normally plethoric and have hemoglobin values around 17 mg/dl. Often delayed cord clamping or positioning the newborn too low or high relative to the placenta will cause plethora or pallor. Twin-to twin transfusions will cause plethora in the recipient and pallor in the donor. Plethora may be present in infants of diabetic mothers, and those with Beckwith-Weidemann syndrome adrenogenital syndrome or thyroid disorders. Pallor is usually due to blood loss (including placental), but also it is important to consider sepsis and severe congenital heart disease (heart failure). Congenital anemia not from blood loss is relatively rare, but one must consider dyserythropoiesis, Blackfan-Diamond syndrome, neonatal Parvovirus B-19 infection and hemolytic disease (alloimmune, autoimmune). Anemia in its severest form may be associated with severe edema (hydrops fetalis) as a consequence of high-output cardiac failure. The chapter on neonatal hematology will supplement this further.

Jaundice

Neonatal jaundice is extremely common and is usually benign and self-limiting such as physiologic (3rd day) jaundice breast-feeding jaundice. These are primarily due to lower levels of UDP glucuronyl transferase in the first days of life and lack of emptying of the colon causing retention of bilirubin and its subsequent enterohepatic re-circulation. All newborns are screened with a serum or trans-cutaneous bilirubin level during the first 24 hours of life. Reliable nomograms have been developed (figure 18) to determine who will be at risk for developing a bilirubin >95 pecentile.

We will discuss causes of jaundice requiring intervention with emphasis on when to suspect and how to identify them. As a general rule, clinically apparent jaundice within the first 24 hr. of life merits closer scrutiny. Also, jaundice appearing after the third day may be significant. If a newborn has other signs including but not limited to fever, tachypnea, pallor, lethargy, vomiting, distention, immediate evaluation is necessary. Usually unconjugated hyperbilirubnemia (see below) will appear with a yellow or orange tinge, whereas conjugated hyperbilirubinemia will appear with a greenish hue.

Simplistically, jaundice is intra-hepatic, hepatic and post hepatic. A normal red blood cell has a lifespan of 120 days, hemolyzes and releases unconjugated bilirubin, which is then circulated through the liver for conjugation to a water-soluble diglucuronide (see GI chapter for further detail). Thus, pre-hepatic jaundice will be unconjugated hyperbilirubinemia, intra-hepatic jaundice may be either conjugated, unconjugated, or both, depending on whether the disorder occurs before or after conjugation. Post hepatic jaundice occurs after conjugation, involves the biliary system from the canaliculi to the larger ducts and is conjugated hyperbilirubinemia.

Pre-hepatic jaundice: This reflects the excessive breakdown of RBC releasing unconjugated bilirubin into the bloodstream. Consider hemolytic causes of excessive RBC breakdown such as innate membrane defects (spherocytosis, elliptocytosis, pyknocytosis, and stomatocytosis). A normal RBC membrane may be vulnerable to breakdown by abnormal enzymes as seen in G6PD, and pyruvate kinase deficiency. Note that hemoglobinopathies such as sickle cell disease do not cause jaundice in the newborn because of the protective effect of fetal hemoglobin. It is important to consider immunologic causes, alloimmune such as Rh, ABO and other minor blood group incompatibility as well as, more rarely, autoimmunity. In maternal autoimmune disease, antibodies may cross the placenta causing temporary symptoms in a newborn. Also bleeding into an enclosed space such as cephalohematoma, intracranial or intramuscular hemorrhage will cause more rapid breakdown and release of RBCs. If a newborn is polycythemic, the excess volume of RBC breakdown will predispose to unconjugated hyperbilirubinemia. Sometimes inadequate intake will prevent passage of bilirubin through the urine and stool. Bilirubin may re-oxidize to unconjugated form (bilirubin oxidase) and cause jaundice. Infants with Down syndrome, infants of diabetic mothers, male infants, infants whose mothers have received oxytocin, gestation <38 weeks, hypothyroidism and Asian infants are more susceptible to prolonged unconjugated hyperbilirubinemia.

Intrahepatic jaundice: This type of jaundice refers to malfunction at the carrier protein step during which time bilirubin transfers into the hepatocyte, the conjugation step during which time UDP diglucuronosyl transferase polarizes the bilirubin molecule to the water-soluble form and the step that releases conjugated bilirubin into the bile canaliculi. Gilbert's syndrome will affect carrier protein function and is associated with higher neonatal bilirubin levels. Absence of conjugating enzyme may be partial in the autosomal dominant form or complete in the lethal autosomal recessive form of Crigler-Najjar syndrome. Breast milk jaundice is presumably due to a steroid compound inhibitor of conjugation in contrast to breast-feeding jaundice which is most likely due to diminished intake as maternal milk supply builds up during the first 3 days of life. Infection, bacterial, viral, or fungal will impact hepatic structure and function. Damaged hepatocytes, especially when disseminated intravascular coagulation is present will produce conjugating enzyme deficiency. Note that intrahepatic jaundice may contain conjugated bilirubin as infection will often damage bile canaliculi as well. Rotor and Dubin Johnson (black pigmented liver) syndromes are due to inability of the hepatocyte to release conjugated bilirubin.

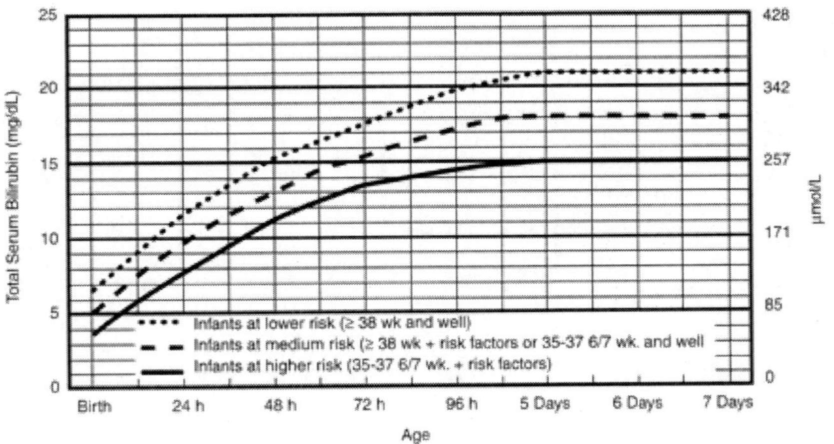

Figure 18. Nomogram for determining use of phototherapy in term newborns.

Post-hepatic jaundice: Disorders of biliary drainage through the smaller ducts up to the common bile duct, cystic duct and gall bladder causes conjugated hyperbilirubinemia. Typically the jaundice persists and may produce a more greenish color to the skin. Other findings such as acholic stools and hepatomegaly may be present. It is critical to address the possibility of biliary atresia first, as prompt diagnosis and early intervention with the Kasai procedure will produce better long-term results. Other causes of conjugated hyperbilirubinemia include congenital paucity of bile ducts, Byler syndrome, inspissated bile syndrome, choledocal cyst, congenital infection (TORCH), bacterial sepsis, neonatal hepatitis and metabolic diseases such as α-1-antitrypsin deficiency, tyrosinemia, and galactosemia and mecomiun ileus secondary to cystic fibrosis.

Management of jaundice: The American Academy of Pediatrics has issued guidelines for the use of phototherapy for jaundice in the otherwise healthy term newborn. This is best described in the nomogram presented in figure 18 (8). Indication for exchange transfusion as per the American Academy of Pediatrics Guidelines of 1999 appears in figure 19.

AAP Guidelines for Phototherapy Treatment

Age, Hours	Consider Phototherapy		Phototherapy		Exchange Transfusion If Intensive Phototherapy Fails		Exchange Transfusion and Intensive Phototherapy	
≤ 24								
25 – 48	≥ 12	(170)	≥ 15	(260)	≥ 20	(340)	≥ 25	(430)
49 – 72	≥ 15	(260)	≥ 18	(310)	≥ 25	(430)	≥ 30	(510)
> 72	≥ 17	(290)	≥ 20	(340)	≥ 25	(430)	≥ 30	(510)

9002110, 9/99

Figure 19. AAP 1999 Guidelines for phototherapy and exchange transfusion.

CONFIRMATORY LABORATORY AND IMAGING

Screening is an integral part of care for all newborns. All screening tests should be sensitive, cost efficient, have a beneficial intervention and have reliable backup tests for positive results. There has been recent rapid expansion of newborn screening. It is incumbent upon the primary care physician to act immediately on any abnormal newborn screen. It is critical to develop systems whereby results are provided quickly and all relevant providers should be able to access this information easily.

We outline laboratory and imaging studies to corroborate diagnostic suspicions based on prenatal history, physical examination and abnormal clinical signs in tables 6, 7 and 8 below.

Table 6. Summary of initial laboratory and imaging based on prenatal history

Prenatal History	Laboratory	Imaging
Maternal infectious:		
Group B strep	CBC, cultures, Urinalysis	Chest x-ray (CXR)
Hepatitis B	Hepatitis panel	Head CT if
TORCH infections	TORCH titers, urine CMV	micro/macrocephaly
HIV infection	cult.	
Herpes Hominis	ELISA studies, Western	
Maternal non-infectious:	Blot	MRI of head
Diabetes	Culture (eye, throat, rectal)	
ITP	LFTs	
Hyper/hypothyroidism		
Drug abuse	Glucose, Hgb, Ca^{++}	
	Platelet count	
Oligohydramnios	T_4, TSH	
Polyhyrdamnios	Drug screen of blood,	GU ultrasound
	urine or meconium	Head CT, CXR, Abd flat
Abnormal prenatal	Urinalysis, BUN,	plate especially if
ultrasound	creatinine	symptomatic
	Glucose Hgb, Ca^{++}	Repeat ultrasound + CT or
		MRI to better delineate
Fetal bradycardia		abnormality
Fetal Tachycardia	Chromosomes if multiple	
	abnormalities	
	EKG Lupus antigens if 3°	
	block	
	EKG, T_4, TSH	

Table 7. Summary of appropriate laboratory and imaging based on initial physical assessment

Physical Finding	Laboratory	Imaging
Large for gestational age	Glucose, Hgb, Ca^{++}	X-ray clavicle if suspect
Small for gestational age	Glucose, TORCH titers,	fracture
	chromosomes (if dysmorphic)	CT of head if suspect TORCH
Dysmorphic features	Chromosome studies	Echocardiogram if suspect
		Down syndrome
Macrocephaly	Chromosomes, toxoplasmosis	CT if suspect hydrocephalus
Microcephaly	titer	CT if >2 SD below mean
Hyper/hypotelorism	Chromosomes, TORCH titers	MRI of head
Blue sclerae	Chromosomes if dysmorphic	Bone series for fractures

Table 7. (Continued)

Physical Finding	Laboratory	Imaging
Enlarged, simple, low set, atretic ears	Chromosomal studies	
Obstructed nares		
Cleft palate	O_2 saturation (Pulse oximetry)	CT of choanal region
Short neck severe torticlollis	Chromosomes if dysmorphic	Swallow study, if necessary X-ray of cervical spines
Web neck	Chromosomes for Turner syndrome	
Heart murmur	Pulse ox, hyperoxia test	EKG, Echochardiogram
Cyanosis	Pulse ox, blood gas, hyperoxia test	CXR, EKG, Echocardiogram
Jaundice	Bilirubin (total and direct), Type and Coombs, CBC, reticulocytes, TSH if severe and persistent, sweat Cl^-, $\alpha 1$ antitrypsin, galactose, tyrosine, if conjugated	HIDA scan if ↑direct bilirubin
Scaphoid abdomen	Basic metabolic panel (BMP)	CXR, Abd flat plate
Abdominal distention	BMP (glucose, electrolytes BUN)	Abd flat plate, Ultrasound or CT
Abdominal mass		
2-vessel umbilical cord		Abdominal ultrasound→CT
Enlarged testicle		Abd ultrasound if dysmorphic
Enlarged painful testicle		Consider ultrasound
Hypospadias		Immediate ultrasound
Hypogonadism		GU ultrasound for anomalies
Micropenis or ambiguous genitalia	BMP, Chromosomes	
	BMP, Chromosomes, DHEA and androgen level, cortisol level, FSH, LH, STH, Prolactin	Pelvic ultrasound or MRI
Virilization	BMP, Chromosomes, 17OH progesterone, ACTH, DOC levels, Androgens, estrogen levels in females	Pelvic ultrasound or MRI
Limb deformities	Chromosomes if dysmorphic	x-rays

Table 8. Summary of laboratory and imaging studies based on key signs

Key sign	Laboratory	Imaging
Hyperthermia	CBC, U/A, CRP, Urine and blood cultures, LP if ill-appearing (sepsis eval) HSV eval (see table 6)	CXR CXR
Hypothermia if symptomatic	As in hyperthermia + glucose, lytes, pH and NH_3 if ill-appearing	CXR
Tachypnea	As in hypothermia	CXR, Echocardiogram if suspect cardiac disease, Head CT if suspect CNS disease
Apnea	As in tachypnea + toxicology studies if suspicious	CXR, Head CT if suspect CNS disease
Vomiting	As in hypothermia	Abd x-ray (air-fluid levels, no gas in rectum, double-bubble of duodenal obstruction),
Irritability/jitteriness	Lytes, BUN, creatinine, glucose, Ca^{++}, PO_4, bilirubin if jaundice, Parathyroid hormone, Chromosome 22 eval if $\downarrow Ca^{++}$	Ultrasound, CT if necessary Head CT if suspect CNS prob,
Seizures	As in irritability/jitteriness, pH, NH_3, TORCH titers. Consider sepsis/meningitis eval if febrile or ill-appearing	Cranial ultrasound, Head CT, EEG
Cyanosis, heart murmur, jaundice	As in Table 7	As in Table 7
Pallor, plethora	CBC	

CONCLUSION

We have outlined an approach to the newborn particularly while in the newborn nursery. We emphasized the importance of taking a thorough and careful history, performing a complete examination and methods of troubleshooting for problems that may occur in the neonatal period. Our goals were to develop the reader's skills to develop a differential diagnosis and subsequent plan of management. We have presented several charts and illustrations for reference, and with repeated usage of this review we hope to inculcate a fund of "pocket knowledge" for health providers in the term newborn nursery.

REFERENCES

[1] Feinberg AN. The term newborn. In: Greydanus DE, Feinberg AN, Patel DR, Homnick DN, eds. The pediatric diagnostic examination. New York: McGraw Hill Medical, 2008:69-110.

[2] Warren JB and Phillipi CA. Care of the well newborn. Pediatr Rev 2012; 33(1):4-18.

[3] Kliegman RM, Stanton BF, St Geme III JW, Schor NF, Behrman RE, eds. Nelson textbook of pediatrics, 19th ed. Philadelphia, PA: Elsevier Saunders, 2011.

[4] American Academy of Pediatrics. Neonatal resuscitation program. URL: http://www2.aap.org/nrp/

[5] Mannino F. Neonatal complications of postterm gestation. J Reprod Med 1988;33(3):271-6.

[6] MacDonald MG, Mullett MD, Seshia MMK, eds. Avery's neonatology: Pathophysiology and management of the newborn, 6th edition. Philadelphia, PA: Lippincott Williams Wilkins, 2005.

[7] Custer JW, Rau RE, eds. The Harriet Lane handbook, 18th ed. Philadelphia, PA: Elsevier/Mosby, 2009:484.

[8] American Academy of Pediatrics. Management of hyperbilirubinemia in the newborn infant 35 or more weeks of gestation. Pediatrics 2004; 114(1):297-316.

[9] Dixon SD, Stein MT. Encounters with children, pediatric behavior and development, fourth ed. Philadelphia, PA: Mosby/Elsevier, 2006.

In: Born into this World: Health Issues
Editors: D. E. Greydanus, A. N. Feinberg et al.
ISBN: 978-1-63321-667-9
© 2014 Nova Science Publishers, Inc.

Chapter 3

THE LATE PRETERM NEWBORN

Geoffrey De Tolve, MD*

Bronson Pediatic Referral Service, Bronson Methodist Hospital,
Kalamazoo, Michigan, United States of America

A selected population of preterm newborns has been receiving increasing attention and recognition over the past decade. Improved standards of prenatal care, successful arrest or delay of preterm labor, and a new generation of well-informed patients have all contributed to a predictable and well-defined decrease in the numbers of early and mid-preterm infants. Coincidentally, if not consequently, increased percentages of late preterm newborns have emerged and these patients have demonstrated significant and specific physiologic differences from their term- and from their early- and mid-preterm colleagues. This review is devoted to a review of the definition, prevalence, short and long term consequences, physiologic differences, and some care and treatment recommendations for this emerging and unique newborn group.

INTRODUCTION

"Late preterm" defines those babies born between 34 0/7 and 36 6/7 weeks' gestation. Engle, Tomashek, and Wallman (1) very appropriately described

---

* Correspondence: Geoffrey De Tolve, MD, Newborn Hospitalist, Bronson Pediatic Referral Service, Bronson Methodist Hospital, 601 John Street, Kalamazoo, Michigan 49007, United States. E-mail: detolveg@bronsonhg.org.

 Geoffrey De Tolve

these newborns collectively as "…A population at risk". The medical literature has exploded with original articles discussing phenomena in these newborns. Of particular interest in recent years are the short and long-term cognitive, intellectual, and social sequelae that these patients experience as they grow and mature (1,2) (see figure 1).

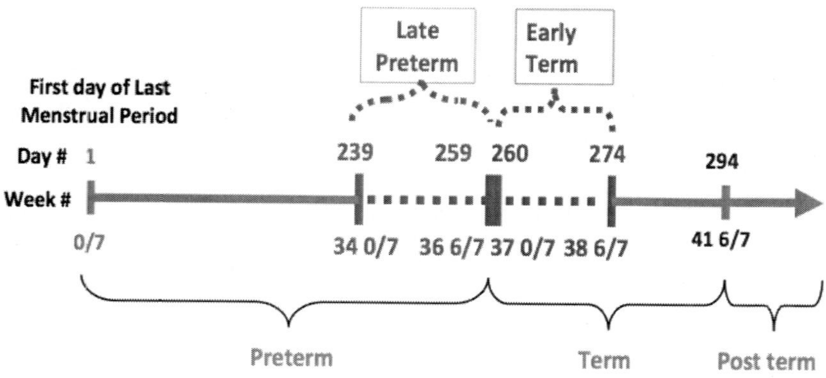

Figure 1. Late Preterm and Early Term definitions.

IDENTIFICATION OF LATE PRETERMS

The gold standard for accurately identifying late preterms remains ultrasonography. "Ultrasound examination results are considered to be consistent with menstrual dates if there is a gestational age agreement within three days by crown-rump length measurement obtained at 6-10 weeks of gestation." In general, ultrasound assessments performed before 20 weeks are highly reliable, but the earlier they are performed, the more accurate (3).

In the event of late, sporadic, or absent prenatal care, the New Ballard score for newborns is accurate in determining gestational age within 1.58 weeks. This scoring system reviews both neuromuscular features as well as physical signs of differing degrees of prematurity (4). It is obtainable at http://www.ballardscore.com

Use this score sheet to assess the gestational maturity of your baby. At the end of the examination the total score determines the gestational maturity in weeks. Figure 2 below is the standard gestational maturation chart. The task of accurately and consistently identifying late preterms is a critical process; indeed, early identification directs a cascade of specific treatment regimens. It is interesting to note that, prior to 1960, by international agreement, all babies were classified as preterm if their birth weight was 2,500 grams or less.

According to Engle, late preterms are physiologically and metabolically immature. As a consequence, these neonates are at greater risk of developing medical complications that result in higher rates of mortality and morbidity during the birth hospitalization. In addition, late preterms have higher rates of hospital readmission during the neonatal period than do term infants (1). Risk factors for readmission include being first born, breast fed at discharge, having a mother who had labor and delivery complications, being a recipient of public assistance at delivery, and also being of Asian or Pacific island descent. In addition, MacBird et al. have found that late preterms are at increased risk of poor health- related outcomes during their birth hospitalization and of increased health care utilization during their entire first year (5).

SCOPE AND INCIDENCE OF LATE PRETERMS

Hamilton found that the rate of late preterm births consistently comprises over 70% of all preterm births in the United States. Although the overall incidence of prematurity has slightly decreased over the past few years, there has occurred a 30% increase of prematurity over the past 20 years-and late preterms accounted for the majority of these. It is noteworthy that the rate of neonatal mortality (death occurring within 0-6 days of life) is nearly 6 times higher than that of term newborns (6). In addition, the risk of late neonatal morbidity (death at 7-27 days of life) is three times higher in late pre term births than for term newborns, and they are twice more likely to die from sudden infant death syndrome than are term infants.

SIGN	SCORE							SIGN SCORE
	-1	0	1	2	3	4	5	
Skin	Sticky, friable, transparent	gelatinous, red, translucent	smooth pink, visible veins	superficial peeling &/or rash, few veins	cracking, pale areas, rare veins	parchment, deep cracking, no vessels	leathery, cracked, wrinkled	
Lanugo	none	sparse	abundant	thinning	bald areas	mostly bald		
Plantar Surface	heel-toe 40-50mm: -1 <40mm: -2	>50 mm no crease	faint red marks	anterior transverse crease only	creases ant. 2/3	creases over entire sole		
Breast	imperceptible	barely perceptible	flat areola no bud	stippled areola 1-2 mm bud	raised areola 3-4 mm bud	full areola 5-10 mm bud		
Eye / Ear	lids fused loosely: -1 tightly: -2	lids open pinna flat stays folded	sl. curved pinna; soft; slow recoil	well-curved pinna; soft but ready recoil	formed & firm instant recoil	thick cartilage ear stiff		
Genitals (Male)	scrotum flat, smooth	scrotum empty, faint rugae	testes in upper canal, rare rugae	testes descending, few rugae	testes down, good rugae	testes pendulous, deep rugae		
Genitals (Female)	clitoris prominent & labia flat	prominent clitoris & small labia minora	prominent clitoris & enlarging minora	majora & minora equally prominent	majora large, minora small	majora cover clitoris & minora		
TOTAL PHYSICAL MATURITY SCORE								

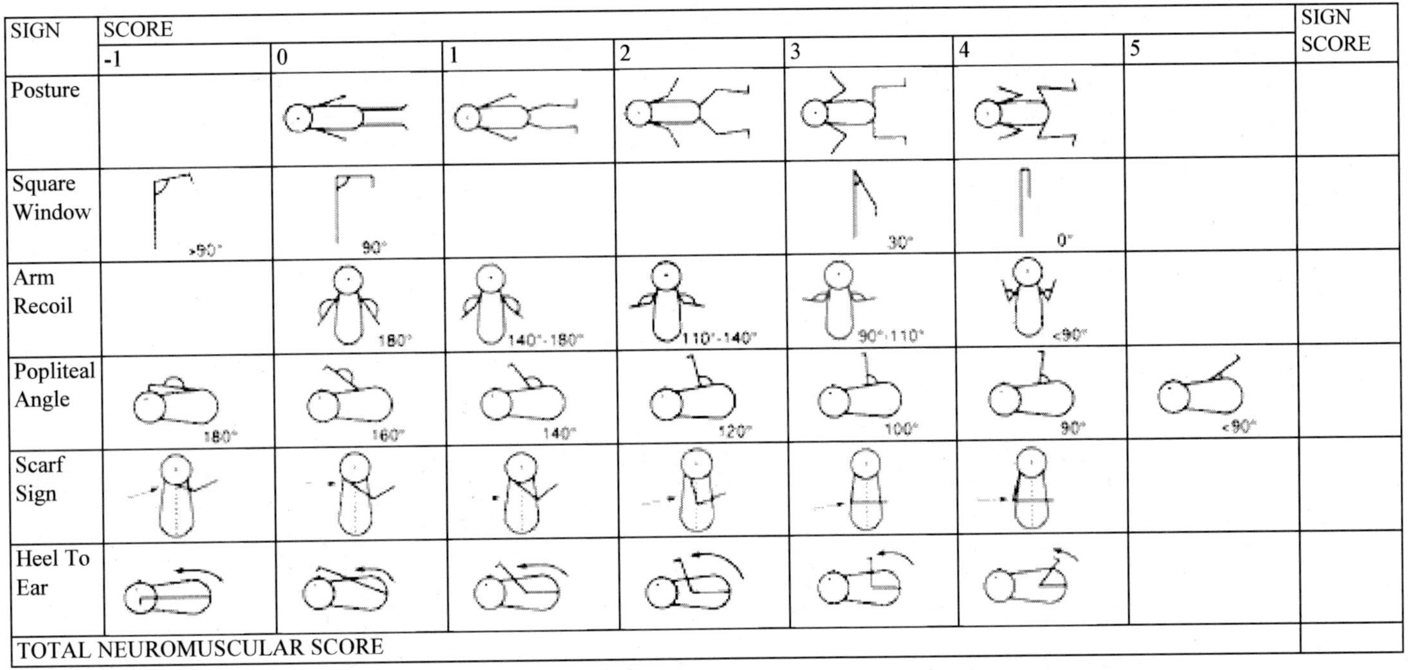

SIGN	SCORE							SIGN SCORE
	-1	0	1	2	3	4	5	
Posture								
Square Window	>90°	90°			30°	0°		
Arm Recoil		180°	140°-180°	110°-140°	90°-110°	<90°		
Popliteal Angle	180°	160°	140°	120°	100°	90°	<90°	
Scarf Sign								
Heel To Ear								
TOTAL NEUROMUSCULAR SCORE								

Figure 2. Chart to assess neuromuscular and physical maturity in newborns of various gestational ages.

NEURODEVELOPMENTAL RISKS

Consider that the fetal brain at 34 weeks weighs only 65% of the term fetal brain. This phenomenon requires a 35% increase in size to attain the size of the term infant's brain. Central nervous system insults related to physiologic risks during this critical time period can deliver long term developmental consequences. The potential for both short and long term cognitive, behavioral, and developmental problems has also emerged as a threat to the health of late preterm newborns. This information is well documented and it continues to be intensively studied and understood. Talge's study in 2010 demonstrated that late preterm births, on the average, are associated with cognitive and socio-emotional problems even after adjusting for important co-variants (7).

PHYSIOLOGIC RISK FACTORS

Multiple physiologic risk factors exist for late preterm infants. We will address concerns in the areas of respiratory, thermoregulatory, metabolic (glycemic control), infections, hyperbilirubinemia and nutritional feeding.

Respiratory

Vital signs and general assessments are initiated immediately after birth, and these continue throughout the newborn hospital stay. Among the most critical of assessments is the respiratory status. Lack of surfactant, airway (integrity) compromise, and poorly developed accessory muscles of respiration are all physiologic components of late preterm infants. Khashu et al (8) have found that late preterm infants have a 4.4 times increased incidence of respiratory distress from a variety of sources. Babies born at 35 weeks have a nine times greater incidence of respiratory distress than term infants. Also, the overall risk for respiratory morbidity is 2-3 times greater before 37 weeks in Caesarean versus vaginally delivered late preterm infants (8).

Tachypnea shortly after birth of any newborn is a normal phenomenon, self-limited, which generally resolves within 1 to 2 hours. Persistent, severe, or progressive tachypnea, hypoxia, retractions, nasal flaring, or grunting may be signs of an intrinsic disease process. Concerns include respiratory distress syndrome, transient tachypnea of the newborn, amniotic fluid or meconium aspiration syndromes. Pulse oximetry, capillary or arterial blood gases, chest x-ray, and a comprehensive physical examination become paramount. Newborn respirations are best counted over a period of 1 full minute.

Careful review of the maternal, prenatal, perinatal delivery history is also critical. Immediate interventions include oxygen administration, the use of a radiant warmer, Doppler blood pressure checks, and continuous careful attention to profusion, tone, activity, and the work of breathing. Infants severely affected based upon their clinical condition may require blood gases, an initial chest radiograph, or a combination of the above may require continuous positive airway pressure (CPAP) or the use of a ventilator.

Thermoregulatory

The immediate perinatal (0-4 hours of life) period calls for creation of a neutral thermal environment. Neutral thermal environment might be defined as that atmosphere in which oxygen consumption is kept at a minimum. The neutral temperature during the first week of life is dependent upon gestational age (and postnatal age), whereas after the first week this parameter depends upon body weight and postnatal age.

Physiologic differences in late preterms include an immature epidermal layer, a higher ratio of body surface to body weight, and poor intrinsic temperature regulating mechanisms. These infants are less effective in generating heat from brown adipose tissue. Careful attention must be made to temperatures every 30 minutes until stable for the first 2 hours, then at least once per shift as recommended. (Normal axillary temperatures consist of 36.5 degrees Centigrade to 37.4 degrees Centigrade or 97.7 degrees Fahrenheit to 99.3 degrees Fahrenheit).

Measures to establish and maintain a neutral thermal environment include use of pre-warmed blankets, a soft cap, a preheated radiant warmer, and kangaroo care. The latter is a long-standing practice that has gained wide acceptance in this country over the past 20 years, with measurable clinical benefits which include:

- Heart rate stabilization
- More regular respirations
- Improved oxygen saturations
- More rapid weight gain

- More successful breast feeding episodes
- Earlier hospital discharges

Hypoglycemia

Wang et al (9) published that low blood sugars occur three times as often in late preterm infants. In fact, blood glucose levels typically decrease in every newborn after birth and reach their nadir at approximately 2-4 hours of life. In the late preterm infant, there are absent low glycogen reserves, decreased gluco-neogenic enzymes, depressed hormonal responses, and slower post-natal increases after reaching the nadir.

In every labor and delivery floor, there exist numerous maternal and neonatal risk factors for hypoglycemia.

Maternal risk factors for hypoglycemia

- Gestational or overt diabetes mellitus
- Pregnancy induced hypertension
- Maternal obesity
- Tocolytics
- Late antipartum IV glucose
- Difficult or prolonged delivery
- Non reassuring fetal heart rate

Neonatal risk factors for hypoglycemia

- Preterm delivery
- Intrauterine growth retardation
- Twin gestation
- 5 minute Apgar less than 7
- Temperature instability
- Sepsis
- Respiratory distress
- Polycythemia

The growing incidence of maternal diet-controlled or insulin-controlled gestational diabetes in particular creates significant risks to the late preterm infant. There exists a transient fetal hyper-insulinemic state and a slow adaptation of the neonatal pancreas to a euglycemic state. Symptoms of neonatal hypoglycemia include poor feeding, hypothermia (not mutually exclusive), an abnormal cry, irritability or lethargy, tremors, excessive jitters, hypotonia, and seizures. Infants can also demonstrate apnea, tachypnea, pallor, cyanosis, and extremes in periodic breathing (9).

Management of hypoglycemia invokes two primary approaches: oral-enteral feedings and IV dextrose. The elegant work of Adamkin, published in February 2011, created algorithms based upon whether the infant is symptomatic or asymptomatic (10). Figure 3 presents an algorithm for management of hypoglycemia. He placed a greater emphasis upon the impact (or not) of feedings upon low blood sugars. However, there remains a need for IV dextrose: in asymptomatic scenarios which include persistently low blood sugars unresponsive to re-feeding or in all symptomatic babies with blood sugars less than 40 mg/dl. The issue of hypoglycemic correction is not an exact science. According to Adamkin, "Current evidence does not support a specific concentration of glucose that can discriminate normal versus abnormal or can potentially result in acute or chronic irreversible neurological damage."

INFECTION: SEPSIS

It is commonly understood that transfer of maternal IgG antibody does not occur efficiently across the placenta until term gestation is reached. In a population-based cohort study of late preterm infants, there was noted a 5.2 times greater risk of suspected or proven sepsis when compared to term infants.

Symptoms of sepsis often mimic those of hypothermia and hypoglycemia. Khashu in 2009 reported that late preterm infants had a higher incidence of hospital readmission when compared to term infants (3.5 versus 2 percent). Approximately one third of these were due to infections in both groups (8).

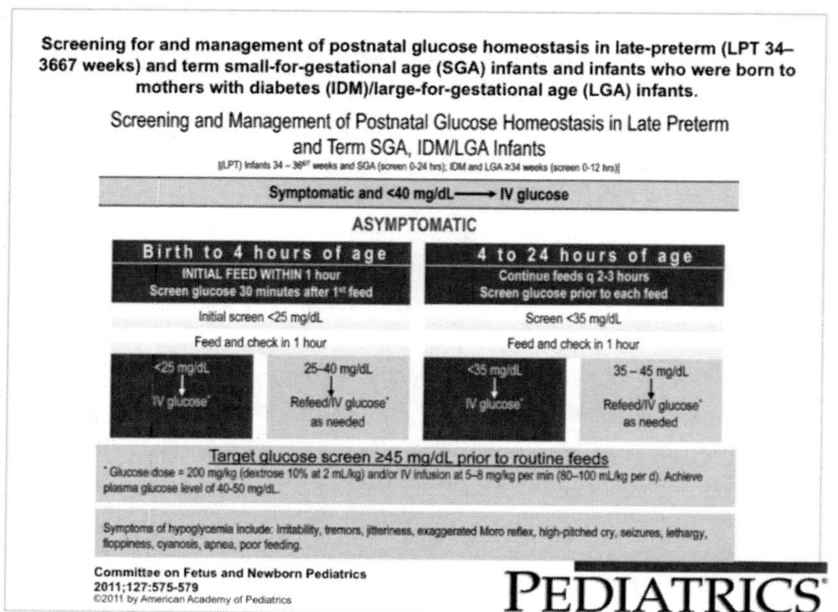

Figure 3. Algorithm for management of hypoglycemia.

Maternal risk factors for sepsis include but are not limited to:

- Prolonged rupture of membranes greater than 18 hours
- Gestation under 37 weeks
- Intra-amniotic infection
- Intra partum fever (100.4 degrees Fahrenheit)
- Young maternal age
- Black race
- Hispanic ethnicity
- Low maternal levels of anticapsular antibodies
- Prior history of Group B Strep disease

Neonatal risk factors for sepsis include:

- Preterm delivery
- Male gender
- Multiple births
- Low birth weight under 2500 grams

- Congenital anomalies
- Stressful delivery
- Black race

Symptoms of sepsis are multifaceted. Features of temperature instability, lethargy, jitteriness, irritability, hypotonia, respiratory distress and hypotension may all represent an early infectious state. Likewise, symptoms of poor perfusion, poor feeding, gastric distension, vomiting/diarrhea, glucose instability, rashes, pustules, petechiae, and jaundice may all represent an early indication of a generalized infectious process.

Close attention to clinical signs and symptoms, review of maternal and neonatal risk factors and clinical intuition must all combine to detect and treat potential infections as early as possible. Figure 4 shows the algorithm published by the American Academy of Pediatrics for the prevention of early-onset group B strep infection in the newborn, adopted from CDC recommendations in 2010 (11).

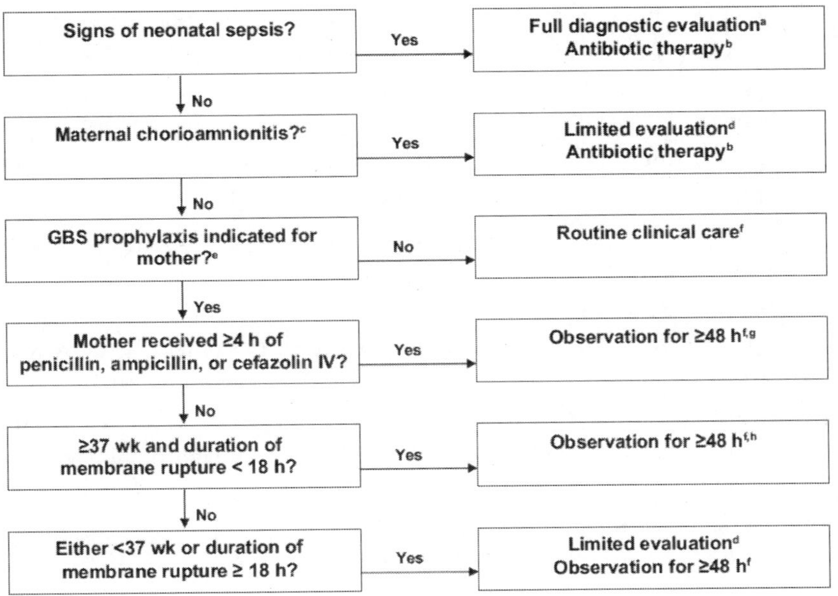

Figure 4. Algorithm for the prevention of early-onset GBS infection in the newborn. (Adapted with permission from Centers for Disease Control and Prevention).

Interpretation of CDC recommendations:

- Full diagnostic evaluation includes a blood culture; CBC count, including white blood cell differential and platelet counts; chest radiograph (if respiratory abnormalities are present); and lumbar puncture (if the patient is stable enough to tolerate procedure and sepsis is suspected).
- Antibiotic therapy should be directed toward the most common causes of neonatal sepsis, including intravenous ampicillin for GBS and coverage for other organisms (including Escherichia coli and other Gram-negative pathogens) and should take into account local antibiotic resistance patterns.
- Consultation with obstetric providers is important in determining the level of clinical suspicion for chorioamnionitis. Chorioamnionitis is diagnosed clinically, and some of the signs are nonspecific.
- Limited evaluation includes blood culture (at birth) and CBC count with differential and platelets (at birth and/or at 6 –12 hours of life).
- GBS prophylaxis is indicated if 1 or more of the following is true: (1) mother is GBS-positive within the preceding 5 weeks; (2) GBS status is unknown and there are 1 or more intrapartum risk factors, including under 37 weeks' gestation, rupture of membranes for > 18 hours, or temperature of >100.4°F (38.0°C); (3) GBS bacteriuria during current pregnancy; or (4) history of a previous infant with GBS disease.
- If signs of sepsis develop, a full diagnostic evaluation should be performed, and antibiotic therapy should be initiated.
- If at >37 weeks' gestation, observation may occur at home after 24 hours if other discharge criteria have been met, there is ready access to medical care, and a person who is able to comply fully with instructions for home observation will be present. If any of these conditions is not met, the infant should be observed in the hospital for at least 48 hours and until discharge criteria have been achieved.
- Some experts recommend a CBC count with differential and platelets at 6 to 12 hours of Age; IV indicates intravenously.

The Canadian Pediatric Society in 2007 stated that "There are no validated, rapid tests that allow the clinician to determine whether an infant with non-specific clinical signs does in fact, have an infection; therefore, ideally, antibiotic therapy should be instituted as quickly as possible in a symptomatic infant (12)."

HYPERBILIRUBINEMIA

Because of delayed maturation, the late preterm infant is deficient in UDP glucuronyl transferase: in fact, there is often less than 1% of adult activity needed to metabolize bilirubin. Also, decreased gastrointestinal motility and poor feeding patterns result in increased gastric re-absorption of bilirubin, further exacerbating this condition. Late preterm infants are twice as likely as term infants to develop hyperbilirubinemia at 5-7 days of life. In addition, the late preterm has a narrower range of safety with regard to bilirubin neurotoxicity, which can develop at an earlier postnatal age than in term infants.

There is a greater risk for hospital readmissions related to jaundice. A review of cases reported to a kernicterus registry found that suboptimal lactation was the most commonly identified contributing factor for severe hyperbilirubinemia and kernicterus in late preterm infants. Visual assessment of jaundice alone is never recommended. However, if jaundice is visually suspected within the first 24 hours, a serum bilirubin level becomes the gold standard for initial assessment. Transcutaneous bilirubins, having emerged largely in the last decade, are best correlated with mid sternum and / or forehead levels. However, it must again be stated here that the gold standard for total bilirubin measurement is the serum total bilirubin.

Current best practice invokes the Bhutani nomogram (13,14). Figures 5 and 6 are the Bhutani nomograms used for term and pre-term infants that assess bilirubin levels by hour of age. In using this graph, the practitioner should:

- Evaluate the total bilirubin levels prior to discharge in all infants, and plot these values on the nomogram.
- Identify those infants at greater risk for hyperbilirubinemia from the history, from feeding criteria, from maternal blood type incompatibilities, and from other risk factors, including bruising, gestational diabetes, breast feeding, and male gender.

                    Geoffrey De Tolve

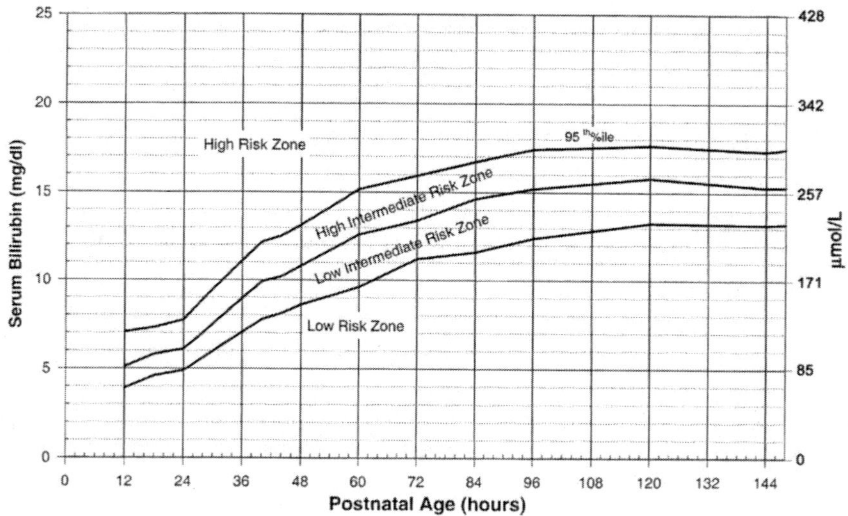

Figure 5. Bhutani nomogram for full term newborns.

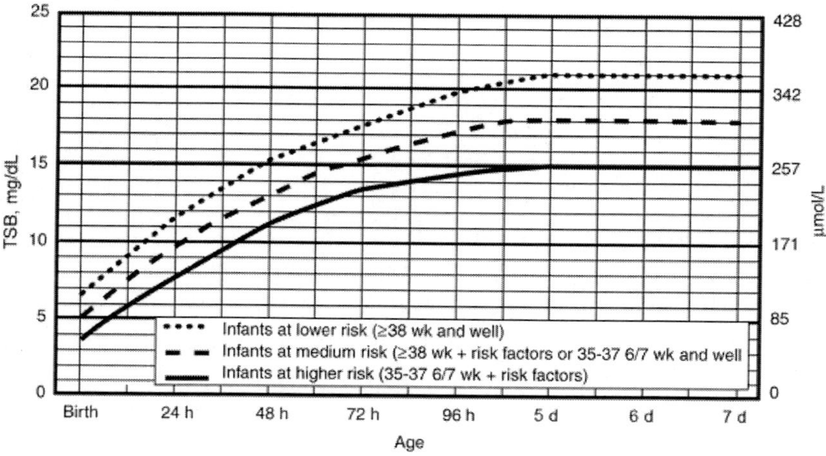

Figure 6. Bhutani nomogram for infants at various gestational ages.

For infants greater than 35 weeks, the practitioner can refer to the following nomogram, which specifically adds prematurity to the other risk factors prior to considering phototherapy) (13,14):

These are guidelines for phototherapy in hospitalized infants ≥35 weeks' gestation. Note that these guidelines are based on limited evidence and that the levels shown are approximations. The guidelines refer to the use of intensive phototherapy, which should be used when the TSB (Total Serum Bilirubin) level reaches or exceeds the line indicated for each category.

- Use total bilirubin. Do not subtract direct-reacting or conjugated bilirubin.
- Risk factors are isoimmune hemolytic disease, G6PD deficiency, asphyxia, significant lethargy, temperature instability, sepsis, acidosis, or an albumin level of <3.0 g/dL (if measured).
- For well infants at 35 to 376/7 weeks' gestation, one can adjust TSB levels for intervention around the medium-risk line. It is an option to intervene at lower TSB levels for infants closer to 35 weeks' gestation and at higher TSB levels for those closer to 376/7 weeks' gestation.
- It is an option to provide conventional phototherapy in the hospital or at home at TSB levels of 2 to 3 mg/dL (35–50 μmol/L) below those shown, but home phototherapy should not be used in any infant with risk factors.

The use of IVIG should be considered in severe instances of iso-hemolytic disease. Exchange transfusions, in more extreme cases, are best performed in the NICU environment, by appropriately trained persons. With any late preterm infant, a close outpatient follow up within 24 to 48 hours, especially when some degree of hyperbilirubinemia is present. In these instances, close communication with the primary care provider is mandatory, regarding current and anticipated future interventions.

FEEDING CHALLENGES IN THE LATE PRETERM NEWBORN

Almost universally, the late preterm infant is subject to some degrees of feeding disorders. Safe and efficient feeding is based upon:

- Oral-motor competence
- Neurobehavioral organization
- Gastrointestinal maturity

Synchronization of these vital functions is usually complete between 36 and 38 weeks. However, exceptions always exist in the practice of medicine. Late preterm infants are different in that they are sleepier, demonstrate less

 Geoffrey De Tolve

stamina, have more difficulty latching on (the breast), exhibit less vigor, and have an immature gastrointestinal function.

Creativity, flexibility, patience, and understanding are key elements needed by the health care team to ensure successful feeding patterns. Some well-known breast feeding interventions include early feeding after birth (when possible), promotion of a goal to feed 10 to 12 times per 24 hours, including through the night, and awakening the infant every 2-4 hours. In addition, facilitate mother's milk production through the use of a breast pump and focus upon positioning as a key component to success.

"Red flags" include a weight loss of greater than 3% per day, or a total of 7 % during the hospital nursery stay. Concerns here arise for infant dehydration, supply and demand issues, feeding frequencies or techniques, and feeding consistency. In a selected number of late preterm infants, feeding struggles or failures in the first 2 to 3 days after birth may, in fact, prompt a longer newborn hospital stay. Such premise may, in the long run, prove more cost-effective, may decrease morbidity and mortality, and may better empower new mothers in their initial breast feeding journey. Such approach may also prevent newborn re-admissions and the logistical and economic implications that may arise in the ever changing health care environment (15).

CONCLUSION

Late preterm infants present many challenges in their care and management. They demonstrate distinct and often predictable physiologic differences which direct a care approach far different from that of their term newborn counterparts. We need to begin to consider all aspects of care for the late preterm infant, and to not consider that they are "near term" and we should not be guided by principles that generally apply to term newborns.

REFERENCES

[1]   Engle A, Tomashek KM, Wallman C, Committee on Fetus and Newborn, American Academy of Pediatrics. Late preterm infants: A Population at Risk. Pediatrics 2007;120:1390-1401.

[2]   Engle WA, Kominlarek MA. Late preterm infants, early term infants, and timing of elective deliveries. Clin Perinatol 2008;35(2):325-41.

[3] Antepartum care. In: American Academy of Pediatrics/American College of Obstetrics and Gynecology. Guidelines for perinatal care, 6th ed. Washington, DC: AAP/ACOG, 2007:83-137.

[4] Ballard JL, Khoury JC, Wedig L. New Ballard Score: expanded to include extremely premature infants. J Pediatrics 1991;119:417-23.

[5] Mac Bird T, Bronstein JM, Hall RW, Lowery CL, Nugent R, Mays GP. Late preterm infants: Birth outcomes and health utilization in the first year. Pediatrics 2010;126(2):e311-9.

[6] Hamilton BE, Martin JA, Ventura SJ. Births: Preliminary data for 2008. Natl Vital Stat Rep 2010;58(16):1-17.

[7] Talge NM, Holzman C, Wang J, Lucia V, Gardiner J, Breslau N. Late-preterm birth and its association with cognitive and socio-emotional outcomes at 6 years of age. Pediatrics 2010;126(6):1124-31.

[8] Khashu M, Narayanan M, Bhargava S, Osiovich H. Perinatal outcomes associated with preterm birth at 33 to 36 weeks' gestation: a population-based cohort study. Pediatrics 2009;123:109-13.

[9] Wang ML, Dorer DJ, Fleming MP, Catlin EA. Clinical Outcomes of near term infants Pediatrics 2004;114(2):372-6.

[10] Adamkin DH. Clinical report. Postnatal glucose homeostasis in late preterm and term infants, Pediatrics 2011;127(3):575-9.

[11] Verani JR1, McGee L, Schrag SJ, Division of Bacterial Diseases, National Center for Immunization and Respiratory Diseases, Centers for Disease Control and Prevention. Prevention of perinatal group B streptococcal disease. MMWR Recomm Rep 2010;59(RR-10):1-36.

[12] Canadian Paediatric Society. Management of the infant at increased risk of sepsis, 2007. URL: http://www.cps.ca/english/statements/FN/FN07-03.pdf

[13] 13. Bhutani VK, Johnson L. Kernicterus in late preterm infants cared for as term healthy infants. Semin Perinatol 2006;30:89-97.

[14] American Academy of Pediatrics. Subcommittee on Hyperbilirubinemia. Management of hyperbilirubinemia in the newborn infant 35 or more weeks of gestation. Pediatrics 2004;114(1):297-316.

[15] Association of Women's Health, Obstetric and Neonatal Nurses. Assessment and care of the late preterm infant. Washington, DC: AWHONN, 2010.

In: Born into this World: Health Issues   ISBN: 978-1-63321-667-9
Editors: D. E. Greydanus, A. N. Feinberg et al.   © 2014 Nova Science Publishers, Inc.

Chapter 4

NEWBORN SCREENING

Arthur N Feinberg[*], *MD, FAAP*
Department of Pediatric and Adolescent Medicine,
Western Michigan University Homer Stryker MD School of Medicine,
Kalamazoo, Michigan, United States of America

ABSTRACT

This review presents the topic of newborn screening from an historical perspective starting with the original Guthrie test for phenylketonuria and chronicles its course of inception to final acceptance. Using this as a springboard we discuss scientific and technical advancements resulting in enhanced screening used today. We update the reader on which tests are employed in which states in the United States. We also discuss criteria for development of screening tests and touch upon several ethical issues such as risks, benefits, costs follow-up and informed consent. Finally we discuss future ethical issues with emphasis on genomics.

---

[*] Correspondence: Professor Arthur N Feinberg, MD, Department of Pediatric and Adolescent Medicine, Western Michigan University Homer Stryker MD School of Medicine, 1000 Oakland Drive, D48G, Kalamazoo, MI 49008-1284 United States. E-mail: arthur.feinberg@med.wmich.edu.

INTRODUCTION

This review discuss newborn screening with emphasis on the history of its emergence and evolution, considerations in developing tests; follow up of results and ethics. The main goal of this review is to provide updates on the science and ethics of screening, to review past ethical issues and to raise many questions about future developments.

HISTORY

The Guthrie test for phenylketonurea (PKU) was developed in 1960. Dr. Robert Guthrie (1916-1995), a microbiologist, who incidentally had a son with intellectual disability and a niece who was diagnosed with PKU, developed a simple and sensitive bacterial inhibition assay to be administered shortly after birth. PKU was first studied as early as the 1930s, and it became more known by the 1960s that those with the condition would have better outcomes if placed on a low phenylalanine diet. However, although it was postulated that the earlier the establishment of the diet, the better the result would be, the only test at the time, the ferric chloride test was unreliable until 6-8 weeks of age.

Although PKU screening is standard and routine today, its early history was not smooth. Dr. Guthrie, in his zeal regarding the condition published a brief report in a letter to the editor at the urging of the National Association for Retarded Children (NARC), who wanted to use this in a 1961 poster child campaign. Although he ultimately published a peer-reviewed study in Pediatrics in 1963, he did fall into disfavor with the academic community because of his previous letter to the editor, his association with NARC, plus his taking the case to parents of retarded children, legislators and the press.

The advent of this test created an upheaval in thinking. Genetic conditions were always considered static not treatable and hopeless. On one end, proponents for the test were hailing its advent as well as looking toward future development of other tests that would greatly improve outcomes of those with metabolic causes of developmental delay. On the other end, vociferous skeptics were concerned about the relative rarity of PKU and that emphasis on it would deflect attention from the vast majority of the mentally retarded who did not have PKU. Those more cautious were concerned about rush to judgment. Some experts claimed that not all individuals with an elevated phenylalanine level were going to be symptomatic and that many would be treated unnecessarily with a very unpalatable diet of Lofenelac. A committee of the American Academy of Pediatrics determined in 1965 that longitudinal developmental data were not adequate to draw any conclusions at this time.

There were concerns about the sensitivity and specificity of the test. It took until 1974 to publish that 10% of infants tested for PKU were missed (either false negative test, not being tested or not finding results) and that only 5.1% with presumably positive tests were confirmed as "classical" PKU, thus having a high false positive rate. However, further studies determined that PKU was not as rare as previously thought, and has an incidence of 1/14000, though rare, nonetheless accounts for a significantly large number of human beings with PKU (1).

A collaborative study ultimately determined that treatment with a low phenylalanine diet as early as possible would be significantly beneficial. However, further studies have determined that those treated still have IQs, though normal, are below those of other family members without PKU. There is also a higher incidence of learning disability, labile emotions and thought disorders. It is not clear whether this is due to imperfection of or occasional lapses in the diet. Ultimately, good cost/benefit analyses determined by 1977 that the benefits of early diagnosis and treatment of PKU outweighed the costs to individuals and to society (2).

Subsequent to PKU testing and its ultimate acceptance, other tests were developed, not without some concerns, but nonetheless implemented. Newborn screening has always been at the discretion of individual states. By the 1970s many, but not all states had a basic panel of tests including Amino acid disorders (PKU) Maple Syrup Urine Disease (MSUD) and endocrine conditions such as Congenital Hypothyroidism (CH) and Congenital Adrenal Hyperplasia (CAH), Hemoglobinopathies (sickle-cell anemia, Hemoglobin C, Thalassemia) and other metabolic disorders such as Galactosemia (GALT), Biotinidase (BIO) deficiency Cystic Fibrosis (CF) and some with Medium Chain Acyl Dehydrogenase Deficiency (MCAD). Also, there was a push in the 1980s for early newborn detection of deafness detected by otoacoustic emissions (OAE), which has now become routine. At present, all 50 states screen mandatorily for the above conditions except hearing screening where 7 states offer, but do not require it and 6 states who offer it to select populations or upon request (3,4). Table 1 below outlines assays used in detecting these basic conditions.

                    Arthur N Feinberg

Table 1. Basic screening tests with follow up tests in parentheses

Condition	Screening Test
PKU	Bacterial Inhibition assay for Phenylalanine (Isoelectric Focusing (IEF), Tandem Mass Spectrometry (MS/MS))
MSUD	Bacterial Inhibition Assay for Leucine, (MS/MS)
CH	Thyroid Stimulating Hormone by immunoassay (lab confirmation)
CAH	17 Hydroxy Progesterone by ELISA, (radioimmunoassay, MS/MS)
GALT	GALT fluorometric study (Beutler analysis, MS/MS)
BIO	Biotinidase, colorimetric assay
MCAD	C6,8,10 Fatty Acids by MS/MS only
Hemoglobin	IEF or High Performance Liquid chromatography (HPLC)
CF	Immunoreactive Trypsinogen (Sweat Chloride test)
Hearing	Oto-acoustic Emissions (Brainstem Auditory Evoked Response)

With the advent of tandem mass spectrometry it is now possible to identify a multitude of metabolic disorders involving fatty acids, organic acids and amino acids. The American College of Medical Genetics has been striving toward developing a uniform policy for screening among the states. At present, all 50 states require testing for 5 fatty acid disorders, 9 organic acid disorders, and 6 amino acid disorders, all designated as "core conditions." There are presently 25 "secondary target conditions" which demonstrate extreme variability in screening among the states. In addition, screening for Critical Congenital Heart Disease (CCHD) with newborn pulse oximetry is mandatory in 6 states and Severe Combined Immunodeficiency (SCID) is mandatory in 7 states at this time. These core conditions are listed in table 2 (5).

Table 2. Core metabolic conditions screened by all 50 states

Fatty acid Disorders
- CUD- Carnitine uptake defect
- LCHAD – Long-chain L-3-hydroxyacyl-CoA dehydrogenase deficiency
- MCAD – Medium chain acyl-CoA dehydrogenase deficiency
- TFP – Trifunctional protein deficiency
- VLCAD – Very long-chain acyl-CoA dehydrogenase deficiency

Organic acid Disorders
- GA-1 – Glutaric academia type I
- HMG – 3-hydroxy 3-methylglutaric aciduria

> - IVA – Isovaleric acidemia
> - 3-MCC – 3-Methylcrotonyl-CoA carboxylase
> - CBL-A,B – Methylmalonic acidemia (Cobolamine/Vitamin B 12 disorders)
> - BKT – Beta ketothiolase deficiency
> - MUT – Methylmalonic acidemia (methylmalonyl-CoA mutase)
> - PROP – Propionic acidemia
> - MCD – Multiple carboxylase deficiency
>
> **Amino acid Disorders**
> - ASA – argininosuccinate aciduria
> - CIT – Cirtullinemia
> - HCY - Homocystinuria
> - MSUD – Maple syrup urine disease
> - PKU – Phenylketonuria
> - TYR-1 – Tyrosinemia type I

CONSIDERATIONS IN DEVELOPING SCREENING TESTS: WHO SHOULD BE SCREENED?

Newborn screening is universal in all states. The conditions are felt to be present in enough people with enough variability among them to justify testing. The prevalence of the conditions may vary, but cost/benefit analyses have proven that as few patients that there may be, the cost of treatment for them outweighs the cost of screening.

However, some conditions are prevalent only in a select population and screening should be limited to that population (targeted screening). As an example Tay-Sachs disease is prevalent in the Ashkenazi Jewish population, thus they should be tested, but not necessarily everyone else. However, there are rare different mutations in other populations (e.g., French-Canadian), which present themselves similarly. Another example is screening for lead poisoning. Currently, high risk children who are more likely to be living in areas with housing stock built before 1950 are identified by Medicaid insurance status. Lead screening is not mandatory in these patients, but health providers are rewarded financially through Medicaid for screening them. With these criteria, a family with means who likes to refurbish old homes or farmhouses would be missed. One might argue to limit screening for sickle-

 Arthur N Feinberg

cell disease to the African-American population, but the rebuttal to that is there is no pure race.

HOW ARE ACCURATE AND RELIABLE SCREENING TESTS DESIGNED?

Any medical test should be carefully evaluated for sensitivity and specificity. As a review, sensitivity represents the ratio of true positive results/all those with the condition. All those with a given condition will either test positive or negative. The negatives would be false, and ideally should be minimized. Specificity represents the ratio of true negative tests/all those without the condition. Similarly, all those without the condition would be either truly negative or falsely positive. In this situation, the false positives (false alarms) should be kept to a minimum (6).

Thus, when one develops a screening test, ideally, the threshold for a positive test should be set at a point where sensitivity of 100% would mean every patient with the condition in question had a positive test. In addition, ideally the threshold selected would also demonstrate a specificity of 100%, meaning that all those without the condition had negative tests.

However, in the real world, each threshold selected will not be perfectly sensitive or specific. Selecting a threshold for a "positive test" too low would identify all those with the condition, but would thus include many without the condition as "positive" (false alarms), thus causing not only anxiety to the patient, but the need to retest. Conversely, setting the threshold too high would take in all the patients who do not have the condition, but would miss many patients who do have it (false negatives). Unfortunately, one cannot calculate sensitivity based on specificity, or vice versa, but there is an empirical relationship between the two, which is very cleverly demonstrated by Receiver-Operator Characteristic Curves (ROC). These were developed in the military to analyze the threshold at which to set radar to detect the presence of mines. The curves are a measurement of the sensitivity (true positive/presence of a mine) on the ordinate from 0-100%. On the abscissa, false alarms, which are actually (1 − specificity), i. e. false positives/absence of a mine, are measured from 0-100%. In plotting sensitivity versus false alarms, if a very large number of detectors (radar, clinicians) generated random yes-no guesses as to whether there are mines, or a given condition, all their true alarms and false alarms plotted on the chart would be all over it. Thus the diagonal line represents a summation of all random guesses. ROC graphs are demonstrated below.

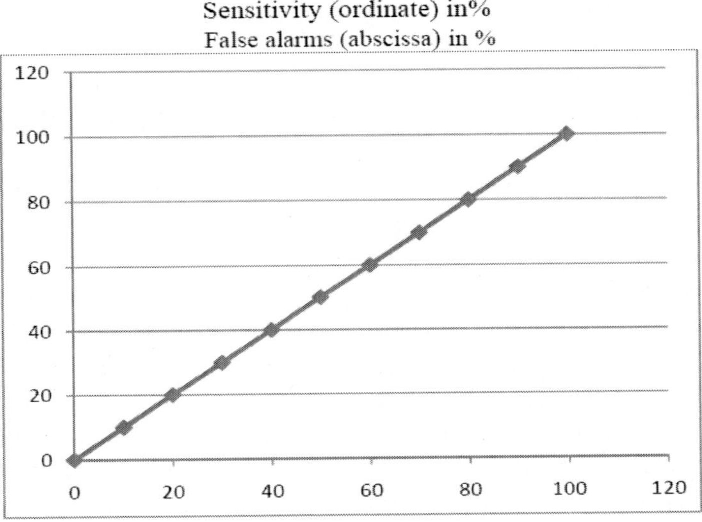

Figure 1. ROC curve demonstrating random distribution.

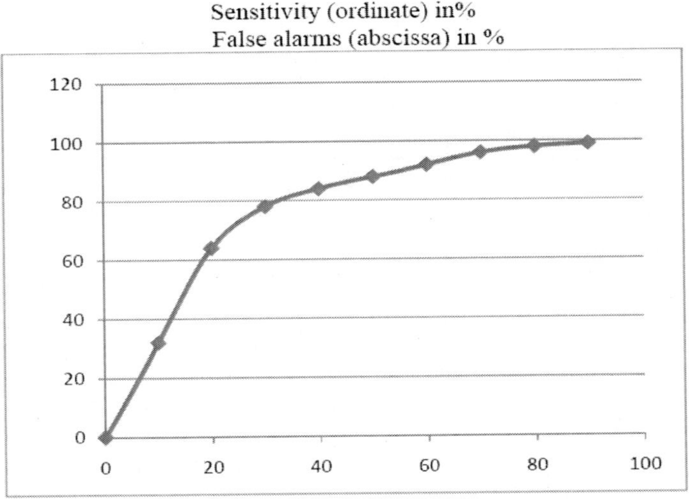

Figure 2. ROC curve demonstrating relationship between sensitivity and false alarms in detecting diabetes mellitus. Varying levels of blood glucose and plotted for sensitivity and false alarms, creating the curve above. (See text for further explanation).

 Arthur N Feinberg

Figure 1 plots false alarms on the abscissa and sensitivity on the ordinate as percentages. The straight line represents a summation of random distribution of yes-no responses. Figure 2 demonstrates a ROC analysis in which a system of detection is chosen. The system would be a test which would have a range of values. Numbers in that range would represent a threshold of detection. Each threshold would be analyzed for true and false positives as well as true and false negatives and plotted accordingly on the chart (7).

As an example, if we are analyzing a system of detecting diabetes using fasting blood glucose in a large population with and without diabetics, we then plot a range of values starting with that which would be the most sensitive (the right-most dot) at 50mg/dl. Each dot moving to the left along the curve represents an increment of 10mg/dl. At each threshold the sensitivity and specificity is calculated and plotted accordingly. The shape of the curve indicates that the threshold with the highest sensitivity and the lowest false alarm rate would be around 110 mg/dl. Each test devised would have a curve of its own. Ideally, the steeper curves with higher points of sensitivity and low false alarms i.e. the largest area under the curve (AUC) would represent the most desirable tests. Note that no test has a plot with 100% sensitivity and 100% specificity (maximal AUC).

FOLLOW UP

Once a test is performed, it is critical to have a system of reporting results. It would be unfortunate if parents or physician of a newborn with an identified condition was not notified in a timely fashion. Many concerns arise as to the possibility of a newborn being cared for by one physician in the hospital and another one at home. How can these results be communicated? Many states have established a central database for immunizations and are now including newborn screens and lead testing. It becomes very simple and it is incumbent upon all health providers to consult this database on all newborns.

Adequate follow up consists of more than merely transmitting a fact to a parent. How much does an individual comprehend what may be potentially shocking news? How can this be measured? Once follow up is ordered, how can it be ensured, especially if time is of the essence? What about all the false positives that have resulted from the screening test? There has to be a definitive backup test that will ensure that the false positives are identified and are truly negative.

In certain circumstances, the same screening test can be used, if reliable (8). As an example, in congenital hypothyroidism, all newborns have a "thyroid surge" at birth with a high output of TSH and T4, so norms at this age are quite high. However, within a week, the levels approach norms for children.

ETHICS

With discovery of increasing possibilities for screening, more thoughtful questions regarding risk, benefit, cost and ethics continued to arise. Should the beneficiaries be individuals, society or both? Once discovered, what is our present knowledge of this possibly rare condition? Can the condition be remediated? How much can it be remediated? Does that matter? Are there means for adequate follow up for those discovered to have the condition at national state and local levels? How can one assure access to the program for those who need it? How costly is this endeavor? Can the results of the screen have a potential for causing collateral harm to the patient (employment, insurability, mental anguish?) Can specimens taken be used for other research? How is confidentiality maintained? Is the patient adequately informed of the risks and benefits? Who will monitor the quality of the program (9)?

What are the risks vs. the benefits?

Benefits consist of detection of a potential serious condition before damage may occur, cause initiation of early treatment and to detect carriers of certain disorders. Risks consist of possible false negative tests resulting in delayed diagnosis, false positive results which may generate anxiety and possible revelation of misattributed paternity, especially when genetic testing is involved. Detection of untreatable conditions could go either way. In some instances some families may be devastated by the revelation; in others, they may want to have the knowledge to prepare them for a very difficult time ahead (10).

Who are the beneficiaries? Are there adverse consequences to non-beneficiaries?

Concerns arise as to the fact that the vast majority citizens with delayed cognition do not have PKU. As a public health measure, would aggressive newborn screening deplete resources to take care of these citizens? If PKU were not curable, resources will also have to be expended to educate them as well (1).

With innovative technology and the marketing thereof, companies who design tests can also be considered collateral beneficiaries. Thus, careful analyses of the validity and reliability of new tests have to be made with no economic incentives causing bias.

What is the present understanding of this condition?

Is there variability among patients with this condition? Can some have a perfectly benign course? How effective is the treatment? Can PKU patients tolerate any phenylalanine at all? What would be considered an acceptable blood level for them? Variant forms of PKU have been discovered which may not require a phenylalanine-free diet. There have been reports of newborns discovered to have high phenylalanine levels whose asymptomatic siblings were tested and had similar levels. Can there be side-effects of the treatment? There were several reports of severe malnutrition in patients treated exclusively with a low phenylalanine formula (11); however, other studies indicate that the small numbers of case reports do not necessarily constitute a major problem (12).

There are major ethical considerations in designing a prospective randomized study treating a not fully-understood condition. Should a non-treated control group be allowed in light of this knowledge, especially if testing a treatment known to be of benefit?

Can the condition be remediated?

Ideally, all conditions identified could be managed, resulting in every patient attaining his/her full potential. However, questions do arise as to whether this is possible. Studies have been published to indicate that appropriate management of patients with such conditions as congenital hypothyroidism and PKU is critical, but nonetheless, even well-treated patients may fall slightly below the norm for developmental milestones (2,13).

THE WILSON AND JUNGNER SCREENING CRITERIA

In 1968 James Maxwell Glover Wilson, Principal Medical Officer at the Ministry of Health in London, England and Gunner Jungner, Chief of the Clinical Chemistry Department of Sahlgren's Hospital in Gothenburg, Sweden developed 10 criteria based on the premise that "in theory, screening is an admirable method of combating disease…(but) in practice there are snags (14)." They have been criticized as being too vague. Many claim that it is difficult to quantify these criteria as they stand, into decision-making tools. Thus, basing national policy on them would be impossible. Also, at the local level, there may be reasons unique to an area or community that would preclude following every principle. Although, not evidence-based, these criteria have stood the test of time.

Other criteria have been developed but when analyzed in a literature search there was a great deal of overlap with the classic Wilson-Jungner criteria. With many questions arising out of the development of the human genome project, plus contemporary notions such as medical ethics, quality control, economics and others, a second set of modified criteria have emerged. In fact, Wilson and Jungner themselves never imagined that their work should become a "gold standard." They stated: "If anywhere we have appeared dogmatic; we hope this may serve to stimulate discussion, since, in the end, real development depends on an exchange of views." Table 3 outlines the original Wilson-Jungner criteria.

Table 3. Classic Wilson Jungner Criteria, 1968

1) The condition sought should be an important health problem.
2) There should be an accepted treatment for patients with recognized disease.
3) Facilities for diagnosis and treatment should be available.
4) There should be a recognizable latent or early symptomatic stage.
5) There should be a suitable test or examination.
6) The test should be acceptable to the population.

Table 3. (Continued)

7) The natural history of the condition, including the development from latent to declared disease should be adequately understood
8) There should be an agreed policy on whom to treat as patients.
9) The cost of case-finding (including diagnosis and treatment of patients diagnosed) should be economically balanced in relation to possible expenditure of medical care as a whole.
10) Case-finding should be a continuing process and not a "once and for all" project.

Table 4. Synthesis of emerging criteria proposed since 1968

• The screening program should respond to a recognized need.
• The objectives of screening should be defined at the outset.
• There should be a defined target population.
• There should be scientific evidence of screening program effectiveness.
• The program should integrate education testing, clinical services and program management.
• There should be quality assurance, with mechanisms to minimize potential risks of screening.
• The program should ensure informed choice, confidentiality and respect for autonomy.
• The program should promote equity and access to screening for the entire target population.
• Program evaluation should be planned from the outset
• The overall benefits of screening should outweigh the harm.

Table 4 consists of criteria that have emerged over the last 40 years in the face of advancing knowledge of genetics with its associated issues such as implications for other family members, uncertainty as to whether having a specific gene will ever produce clinical signs and symptoms, emerging reproductive options. Other significant changes in the landscape of society have included increased consumerism, the shift away from paternalism towards informed consent, evidence-based medicine, case management for cost effectiveness, quality assurance and accountability. Recent analyses of these maintain that the original criteria still stand firm and that there should always be ongoing modifications and development of assessment tools (15).

Arguments have arisen as to whether an irremediable condition should be screened. This arises more with pre-natal and targeted screening. Although there is not direct benefit to the individual being screened, should other family members be considered? As an example, Tay-Sachs disease is not treatable, but would a family benefit from advanced knowledge that it is coming? What about other conditions such as Huntington's chorea? It is not remediable, but would run a much longer course and appear later than Tay-Sachs disease. Some may or may not desire to have knowledge of impending conditions (16).

ISSUES FOR THE FUTURE

With the advent of genetic testing, many more ethical questions arise. A multitude of conditions can now be identified and questions have arisen as to whether society is prepared to support all these patients, both economically and logistically. There are definite risks for the proband identified with a genetic condition: bias, discrimination, stigma, anxiety and economic losses (jobs and insurance). It is not clear whether an individual with a given gene will ever manifest clinical signs and symptoms.

As there is a whole pedigree involved, there always has to be consideration given to other members of this pedigree. Should they know? Who should tell them? Paramount is the consideration of privacy and confidentiality. It is now possible to collect spots of blood and analyze the genomes of individuals or populations. There is a potential for research, which can be valuable. However, if a genetic condition is identified, should the subject be re-contacted? What about other family members who may be affected? Would the subjects want to know this information?

At present, the following is considered basic to informed consent, although there is still variation among individual states (17).

- The purpose of the research, in lay language
- How the specimens will be stored and who will have access to them or to the information contained
- Whether the subjects will be re-contacted later with their individual results or any information about the study
- Whether the samples or genetic information have a code that can be linked to the identity of individual subjects. If a link to identifiers is retained, the sample/information is not anonymous

- Whether the researchers will use specimens to develop commercial products or assays, and whether the subject will be able to share any financial gain from these products
- Whether the researchers plan to conduct future testing of these samples
- Whether samples may be used for other research studies including those that may have a different focus.

Most debate regarding newborn screening centers on expanded newborn screening in the genomic era. The following is a summary of both sides of the debate regarding this (16).

Pro

This is a significant step toward the attainment of personalized medicine. If an individual has the knowledge of his/her genetic susceptibilities, he/she will be able to take steps to reduce risk by increased surveillance, lifestyle modifications, diet or drug therapy. Pediatricians could be of most help as they may have this knowledge of the patient and tailor care and counseling to that individual at an early age as they are developing their lifestyles.

Development of a world biogenetic databank would be of great value to research and develop better understanding of very rare medical conditions. Although the stigma of being labeled with a genetic predisposition is well known, presumably, with all individuals as part of the biobank, the stigma will be diluted with each member feeling part of it. The biobank can be viewed as a lottery. Each genetic predisposition is merely that, not an indicator of clinical presentation or severity. All members will have their share of many of these predispositions, and therefore, unlike the typical lottery, there will be no "winners" or "losers", per se. There would be a feeling of "we're all in this together"

Studies have shown an increasing trend toward consumerism. Simply, more individuals want to know these facts. This is particularly true of parents regarding genetic conditions in their children, so they may provide better support in a more timely fashion. Furthermore, the concept of support can extend beyond the immediate family to enhancing support and advocacy groups that have impact on future public policy.

Con

With the emergence of this vast amount of genetic data, huge infrastructures need to be built to assess outcomes and counsel and support individuals. It is still not clear as to whether there would be any change in outcome with advanced knowledge of an impending medical condition. As an example, Duchenne's muscular dystrophy (DMD) may not become clinically apparent for years. Aside from the anxiety generated, during the latency period there is always the potential of parents seeking deleterious treatments, unbeknownst to them.

Who is the true "owner" of this genetic information? Is it the parent? Is it the child? Can a child fully understand the ramifications? Is there true informed consent so that even an adult can fully appreciate the ramifications? As with true informed consent, any adult should have the opportunity to opt out. This would not be possible with mandatory mass screening.

Newborn screening is bound to extend to prenatal screening. Helping families make future reproductive decisions based on prenatal genetic screening has often been touted as a benefit. This may be applicable for conditions that have guaranteed manifestations that are untreatable and lethal such as Tay-Sachs disease and Huntington's chorea. However, the vast majority of inheritable conditions will have variable penetrance with many degrees of disability. If one child has disabilities and parents decide to terminate any future pregnancies "just like him" what message does it send to that child? Are we basing the worth of an individual on his/her genetic endowment?

Are genes the "be-all-and end-all?" The field of epigenetics has demonstrated the interaction with genes and the environment can be significant. Will genetic screening extend itself to genetic variants which may well be in the normal range? Are we returning to the old failed world of eugenics, and trying once again to create a master race?

NEWBORN SCREENING FOR SPECIAL CARE INFANTS

Premature, small-for-dates and sick newborns present special challenges for newborn screening, mainly because there are many potentially confounding variables at play due to medical conditions and treatments. Presently there is a paucity of research on the interplay of these factors; thus practices are developed by consensus rather than by evidence-based data. It is known that

2-10% of newborn screening specimens are returned as "abnormal" or "insufficient", and of all abnormal and insufficient collections 10-40% of them originate from neonatal special care units.

Instead of presenting recommendations for screening of special care newborns, we will provide questions in need of answers. Guiding principles often center on such practical aspects as limitations of newborn blood supply and their present state of vulnerability and fragility. Primary considerations in screening NICU babies include maternal conditions which may have predisposed to premature delivery, prematurity, low birth weight or illness in and of themselves and the effect of treatment on screening results.

We present below various times of screening with their advantages and disadvantages developed by the CLSI (Clinical and Laboratory Standards Institute).

Screening upon admission

Advantages: Known to be reliable for abnormal hemoglobins, GALT and biotinidase deficiency. Although little is known about disorders of fatty acid oxidation (FAO) in prematures, an initial screen would provide a "baseline" value. Illness and stress may make it easier to detect FAO disorders. Making admission screening a "standard" would increase the chance of capturing more newborns.

Disadvantages: There are known false positive and false negative results for TSH, OHP (17 hydroxyprogesterone) and IRT (immunoreactive trypsinogen).

Screen repeat at 72 hours

Advantages: Demonstrated reliability for congenital hypothyroidism (thyroid origin) and CAH. It is reliable for aminoacidopathies unless parenteral nutrition is being administered.

Disadvantages: Masking due to parenteral nutrition in carnitine disorders as well.

Rescreen at 28 days or upon NICU discharge

Advantages: By this point the thyroid has matured to term newborn levels. Usually resolves previous false positive screens. Longer waiting time will allow interventions to "get out of the newborn's system." Disadvantages: extra cost.

Newborn hearing screening should be performed by one month of age if possible. Keep in mind that neonatal conditions such as cytomegalovirus infections and neonatal treatment with aminoglycosides may have ongoing effects on hearing, even after NICU discharge.

SUMMARY

We have presented an update on newborn screening techniques and reviewed its history and evolution.

We discussed the risks versus the benefits of neonatal screening and presented an analysis of effectiveness of screening based on sensitivity and specificity. We outlined appropriate usage of screening and reviewed ethical issues in neonatal screening, past, present and future.

REFERENCES

[1]   Paul DP. The history of newborn phenylketonuria screening in the US. In: Holtzman NA, Watson MS, eds. Promoting safe and effective genetic testing in the United States. Bethesda, MD: National Human Genome Research Institute, 1997.

[2]   Beasley MC, Costello PM, Smith I. Outcome of treatment in young adults with phenylketonuria detected by routine neonatal screening between 1964 and 1971. Q J Med 1993;87(3):155-80.

[3]   Clague A, Thomas A. Neonatal biochemical screening for disease. Clin Chim Acta 2002;315(1-2): 99-110.

[4]   Levy PA. An overview of newborn screening. J Dev Behav Pediatr 2010; 31(7):622-31.

[5]   Kaye CI, Accurso F, La Franchi S, Lane PA, Northup H, Pang S, et al. Introduction to the newborn screening fact sheets. Pediatrics 2006; 118(3):1304-12.

[6]   Carvajal DN, Rowe PC. Sensitivity, specificity, predictive values and likelihood ratios. Pediatr Rev 2010;31(12):511-3.

[7]   Park SH, Goo JM, Jo CH. Receiver operating characteristic (ROC) curve: Practical review for radiologists. Korean J Radiol 2004;5(1): 11-8.

[8]   American Academy of Pediatrics Newborn Screening Authoring Committee. Newborn screening expands: Recommendations for pediatricians and medical homes. Implications for the system. Pediatrics 2008;121(1):192-217.

[9]   Levy HL. Newborn screening conditions: what we know, what we do not know and how will we know it? Genet Med 2010;12(Suppl 2):S213-4.

[10]   Bailey Jr. DB, Skinner D, Warren SF. Newborn screening for developmental disabilities: Reframing presumptive benefit. Am J Pub Health 2005;95:1889-93.

[11]   Botkin JR, Clayton EW, Fost NC, Burke W, Murray TH, Baily MA, et al. Newborn screening technology: Proceed with caution. Pediatrics 2006;117(5):1793-9.

[12]   Brosco JP, Sanders LM, Seider MI, Dunn AC. Adverse outcomes of early newborn screening programs for phenylketonuria. Pediatrics 2008;122(1):192-7.

[13]   Rose SR. Update of newborn screening and therapy for congenital hypothyroidism. Pediatrics 2006;117(6): 2290-2315.

[14]   Wilson JM, Jungner YG. Principles and practice of mass screening for disease. Bol Oficina Sanit Panam 1968;65:281-3.

[15]   Andermann A, Blancquaert I, Beauchamp S, Dery V. Revisiting Wilson and Jungner in the genomic age: A review of screening criteria over the past 40 yearts. Bull World Health Organ 2008;86:317-9.

[16]   Schulman A. The future of newborn screening: Clouds on the horizon? Washington, DC: President's Council Bioethics, 2008.

[17]   Goodman K. Biomedical 101 refresher course. Genetics research. Miami, FL: CITI Collaborative Institutional Training Initiative, 2012.

In: Born into this World: Health Issues   ISBN: 978-1-63321-667-9
Editors: D. E. Greydanus, A. N. Feinberg et al.   © 2014 Nova Science Publishers, Inc.

Chapter 5

RESUSCITATION

Vinay N Reddy*, MD
Department of Pediatric and Adolescent Medicine,
Western Michigan University,
Homer Stryker M.D. School of Medicine,
Kalamazoo, MI, United States of America

ABSTRACT

Resuscitation of newborn infants has changed over time and national standards have resulted in trained staff, but asphyxia is still the cause of death for many infants dying in the neonatal period. A major change occurred in 2011 with the publication of the 6th edition of the American Academy of Pediatrics/American Heart Association "Textbook of Neonatal Resuscitation". Prior to that time; most courses followed a lecture-demonstration-practice-test format, but now, we leave most of the didactics to the students themselves -- students are required to take the examination, on line, before starting the practical segment of the course -- and, although we still expect near-perfection with individual skills, the main part of the course consists of one or more simulated resuscitations in which a group of students conduct the resuscitation under the instructor's gaze, and then are debriefed with the instructor.

---

* Correspondence: Vinay N Reddy, MD, Department of Pediatric and Adolescent Medicine, Western Michigan University Homer Stryker MD School of Medicine, 1000 Oakland Drive, D48G, Kalamazoo, MI 49008-1284, United States. E-mail: vinay.reddy@med.wmich.edu.

                    Vinay N Reddy

INTRODUCTION

Until the late 1980s, resuscitation of newborn infants, especially at delivery, was not particularly systematic. Neither was training for professionals in neonatal resuscitation -- although national standards for adult cardiopulmonary resuscitation, first recommended by the National Academy of Sciences in 1966, had resulted in many trained resuscitators (including lay people) by the early 1980s. Unfortunately, asphyxia at birth is the cause of death for almost one out of four infants who die in the neonatal period.

In 1978, the American Heart Association (AHA) Committee on Emergency Cardiac Care established a committee to develop standards and procedures for resuscitation of children, and the AHA and the American Academy of Pediatrics (AAP) began to develop a training program in neonatal resuscitation. The Neonatal Resuscitation Program's (NRP) first courses, and the first edition of the AAP Textbook of Neonatal Resuscitation, debuted in 1987-1988, and training based on the textbook spread through the late 1980s and early 1990s. Training and certification in neonatal resuscitation is now a standard of care for physicians, nurse practitioners, and respiratory therapists who attend deliveries -- a far cry, thankfully, from the days when residents performed their first resuscitations on babies instead of plastic manikins.

This review is intended as an overview of current practice guidelines in neonatal resuscitation, with additional comments on the evolution of current standards. It is not intended as a complete guide to neonatal resuscitation; if it is part of your practice you are well-advised to take the NRP course, and to retake it at the prescribed two-year intervals.

THE PHYSIOLOGY OF BIRTH TRANSITION

The most important change at the birth of an infant is the switching of the baby's oxygen source. Throughout gestation in utero, oxygen is provided from the mother's lungs: her arterial blood releases oxygen in the placenta which is then taken up by the baby's umbilical blood. The umbilical venous blood has a higher pO_2 than anywhere else in the fetus; oxygenated umbilical blood enters the right side of the heart, having mixed with low-oxygen blood returning from other organs. Little of the pulmonary blood output enters the pulmonary vasculature, which has a resistance much higher than after birth.

Instead, the bulk of right-ventricle output passes from the right ventricle, through the ductus arteriosus, and into the aorta to be mixed with blood pumped by the left ventricles. Systemic venous blood enters the right atrium, but some of this blood passes through the foramen ovale to the left atrium and eventually is mixed with the (relatively little) pulmonary output. To use an electrical analogue: the ventricles are pumping in parallel in utero.

When the infant takes its first breath, the pulmonary air passages are expanded by inspired air. This reduces the pulmonary vascular resistance, and thus the right-ventricle input and output blood pressures, considerably. The foramen ovale is a one-way valve: blood can pass from right to left, but not from left to right. Once a pulmonary pressure has dropped, the foramen closes and stays closed. In most people, the valve flap of the foramen ovale eventually becomes part of the atrial septum and does not open again. With some people, however, the foramen ovale flap never completely closes. This is not a problem in childhood, unless pulmonary pressures become greater then systemic pressures, which is very rare. However, closure is recommended also because of the possibility of emboli.

In addition, once pulmonary pressures have fallen, blood flow through the pulmonary vasculature increases considerably, and flow through the ductus arteriosus decreases. The ductus blood is now much more oxygenated than prior to birth and the added oxygen causes the ductus to constrict and further decreases flow. Usually, within 12-24 hours the ductus closes permanently. Once the ductus arteriosus and the foramen ovale are closed, the right heart pumps blood only from the systemic veins into the pulmonary arteries, and the left heart pumps blood almost exclusively from the pulmonary veins into the systemic arteries. The bronchial blood vessels are fed blood from the left heart through the systemic arteries, but a small part of the bronchial blood flows into the pulmonary veins and from there to the left side of the heart; this enables the circulatory system to maintain proper amounts of pulmonary and systemic volumes and flow rates even if other mechanisms fail.

THE PERILS OF BIRTH TRANSITION

Many infants have been born through human history with only a low proportion of them dying during or shortly after birth. This proportion has become smaller as we have learned how mothers, infants, and the processes of gestation and delivery work and have invented therapy that can help the infant come to term, but it has never become zero.

Infants may have problems before labor begins, during labor, and/or after delivery. Problems before and during labor are most often caused by decreased blood flow, either in the uterine circulation or in the placental/fetal circulation, which results in hypoxygenation of the fetus. The first sign of this can be deceleration, or slowing, of the fetal heart rate, and is treated initially by improving oxygenation, either by changing the mother's position to relieve pressure on uterine and placental vessels or administering supplemental oxygen to the mother.

Problems after delivery are also due to inadequate oxygenation, but at that point hypoxygenation is most often due to problems in the infant's respiratory tract. Inadequate lung ventilation may occur when the infant cannot clear enough fluid from the alveoli with the initial breaths, or when particulates such as meconium clog the bronchial tree. Hypoperfusion, whether by hypoxia, ischemia, or blood loss, leads to impaired cardiac function (contractility and/or bradycardia) and subsequent hypotension. Pulmonary arterioles normally dilate with the infant's first few breaths and oxygen intake.

Persistent pulmonary hypertension of the newborn (PPHN) can be caused by inability to aerate enough of the bronchial tree for the infant to self-oxygenate, and/or by lack of available oxygen before or during delivery. Either of these can result in impaired pulmonary perfusion, as can persistent pulmonary arteriolar constriction which may be present even after apparently complete lung aeration.

Newborn infants usually inhale air vigorously and immediately upon delivery. This increases air pressure in the lungs, which helps inspiration of oxygen and absorption of lung fluid into the circulation. Pulmonary arterioles relax with higher oxygen exposure, thus increasing pulmonary blood flow. If immediate ventilation does not occur, continued hypoperfusion and fluid retention in the lungs will prevent systemic oxygenation of tissues and cause constrictions of arterioles in the kidneys, gastrointestinal tract (especially the small intestine), and muscles as well as skin. The body will attempt to preserve cerebral and cardiac function by diverting a larger share of cardiac output to those two systems, but if the infant is starved of oxygen for long enough cardiac function, and blood flow and pressure to all organs, fall. This can result in damage to organs, including the brain, and ultimately to death.

SIGNS OF COMPROMISE IN THE NEWBORN INFANT

The entire course of evolving compromise in a newborn infant goes through four stages:

- An initial period of rapid regular breathing.
- A period of primary apnea, without breathing or gasping.
- A period of gasping and irregular breaths.
- A period of secondary apnea, also without breathing or gasping but not followed by spontaneous breathing.

Unfortunately, resuscitating providers are rarely able to observe all four stages, and it is not uncommon for the delivering provider to hand over an apneic baby. It is also not uncommon for the comprising event to have occurred during, or even before, labor. Thus with an apneic infant, one cannot determine by physical findings alone if the apnea is primary or secondary. The only difference is that a baby in primary apnea is likely to begin breathing again immediately after stimulation, while a baby in secondary apnea will not start breathing and thus will need immediate respiratory assistance.

Heart rate may be normal initially, but falls markedly at the beginning of primary apnea, and continues to fall at a lower rate thereafter. Blood pressure tends to remain at normal levels until secondary apnea begins unless the infant has lost blood, in which case blood pressure may drop earlier.

THE FLOW OF NEONATAL RESUSCITATION PROCEDURES

The NRP has developed, and has regularly reviewed and revised, an algorithm for the assessment and resuscitation of the newborn infant. In the 6th edition of the NRP textbook (2) the algorithm is in the form of a flow diagram showing assessments of the infant at each stage of the resuscitation, as well as measures to be taken depending on the findings at each assessment. Caregivers who regularly attend deliveries usually have the algorithm committed to memory -- and should. The rapidity of intrapartum changes in an infant does not leave the resuscitators time to spend looking up the answers in the midst of the resuscitation.

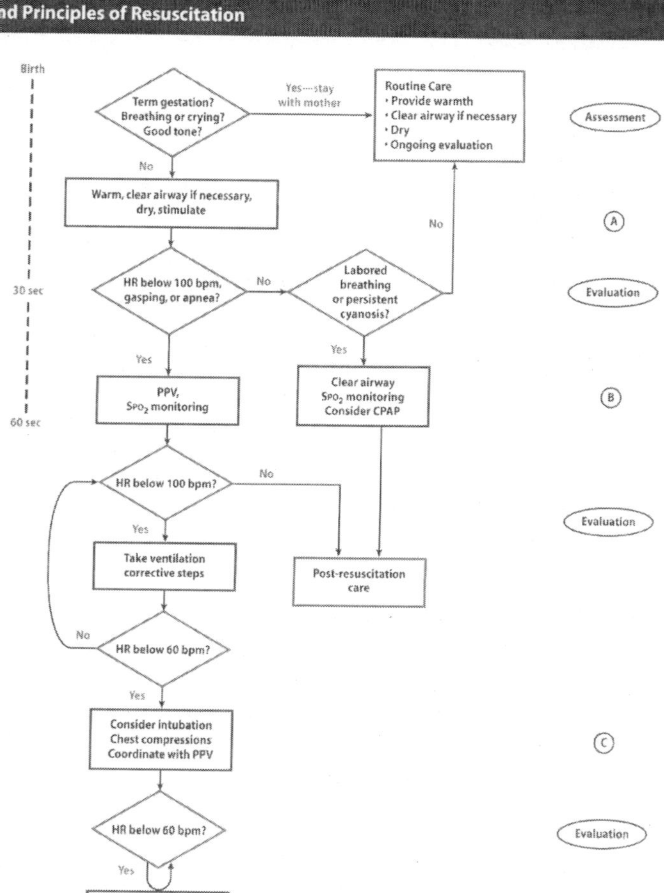

Figure 1. Algorithm for neonatal resuscitation.

The algorithm follows the classic A-B-C's of resuscitation (see figure 1). Before the baby is delivered, the resuscitation team should be briefed on pregnancy and labor problems. As soon as the baby is in its care (usually a few seconds after birth), the sequence of event will be as follows:

Airway

Once receiving the baby, keep it warm -- this can be by skin-to-skin contact with the mother, but an infant that was born prematurely, is not breathing or crying well, and/or is hypotonic, should be placed on a resuscitation table with a radiant warmer on its back or side. Position the head so that the airway is open (remember that, unlike adults, hyperextension of the neck can occlude the infant's airway as much as flexion can), and remove any fluids or particulate material that may obstruct the airway and impair respiration.

If there is visible meconium on the skin or in the nose or mouth, and if the baby is not vigorous, the trachea should be suctioned through a properly-placed endotracheal tube. As recently as the late 1980s, DeLee catheters -- catheters connected to the vacuum source by a trap -- were used to suction meconium-stained fluid from the airway, with vacuum often being provided by the resuscitator's lungs. This method should not be used except in the direst of circumstances. Endotracheal tubes are slightly stiffer, and are easier to place properly, than ordinary catheters, including DeLees.

As for the vacuum source: the trap in a DeLee catheter does not necessarily prevent fluid and particulates from entering the source, a very unpleasant experience for the one who is providing suction. In the past intubation was performed for airway suctioning whenever meconium was found in the amniotic fluid, unless the infant was sufficiently vigorous to prevent the resuscitator from intubating. Since then, it has been found that meconium in the oropharynx is not dangerous as long as the baby is vigorous. However, trainees now perform intubations much less frequently now than in the 20th century. Although good for infants overall, this also leaves trainees with much less practice of, and less comfortable with, neonatal intubation.

Evaluate the infant during and immediately after these initial steps, which you should be able to complete in 30 seconds or less, and ascertain heart rate and respiratory function in this time as well.

Breathing

If the infant is bradycardic (in this circumstance, a heart rate of less than 100 beats/minute) and/or apneic, begin positive-pressure ventilation (PPV). This is usually performed at first with a mask, but intubation may be needed especially if mask ventilation is poor. An infant who is breathing but in respiratory distress -- often premature infants who may have insufficient lung surfactant -- may need continuous positive airway pressure (CPAP) to help keep the alveoli open and increase the lungs' ability to exchange oxygen and CO_2.

In the past 100% oxygen, with or without intubation, was commonly used in neonatal resuscitations. However, studies over the last decade have shown that an infant's oxygen saturation may remain low for several minutes after birth, (preductal SpO_2 usually reaches 85-95% by about 10 minutes post-partum) with no short- or long-term adverse sequelae. Other studies have demonstrated associations between even relatively low/brief increases in oxygen supplied during resuscitation and later increased incidence of certain diseases, including retinopathy of premature (originally described in a term newborn) and acute lymphoblastic leukemia.

If assistance with breathing is required, SpO_2 should be measured with an oximeter to determine the proper amount of supplemental oxygen during the resuscitation, and oxygen concentration should be adjusted based on pulse oximetry to the minimum level needed to support the infant. The oximeter detector should be placed somewhere on the right arm; with this, the oximeter will show preductal SpO_2, which is about the same as SpO_2 in blood flowing to essential organs (i.e. heart muscle and brain) even in the presence of shunting through cardiac anomalies. Postductal placement of the oximeter detector may show abnormally low SpO_2, especially since the ductus arteriosus remains patent for several hours after delivery. This step should also be performed in about 30 seconds. The infant's ventilation must be reevaluated at that time, and further measures taken if ventilation is still poor before you can assess and support circulation.

Circulation

If the infant's heart rate is still low (60/minute of less), circulation must be supported with chest compressions. Since it is difficult to provide effective chest compressions and ventilation at the same time, an infant at this stage should be intubated to improve lung expansion if it has not already been done. Compressions should be performed until the infant's heart rate is greater than 60/minute, and should be synchronized with ventilation so that air exchange is not compromised by the compressions, even if the infant has been intubated (three compressions, followed by one breath, all in two seconds, giving the infant 90 compressions and 30 breaths per minute).

Once the infant's heart rate is over 60/minute compressions should be stopped, but ventilation should continue until the heart rate is over 100/minute and can and should be performed more frequently if compressions are held. A bradycardic infant may need over 45 seconds of compressions to restore coronary perfusion; thus, once compressions are stared, they should be administered for at least 45-60 seconds before stopping briefly to assess the heart rate.

Drugs

When the NRP began, there were five drugs recommended for use in resuscitations. Three of these have since lost their place. Sodium bicarbonate is still used to treat metabolic acidosis and dopamine is still used in cases of hypotension or otherwise poor cardiac output, but these are now used mainly after the acute resuscitation. Naloxone is used to antagonize opiates, sometimes given to the mother therapeutically but sometimes exposed to the infant by substance abuse, but is also now used after initial resuscitation. They were not used very frequently to begin with: in fact, use of medications in neonatal resuscitation has always been rather rare.

A drug still used in resuscitation is epinephrine, a relatively non-selective catecholamine which increases both heart rate and contractility, and also induces peripheral vasoconstriction. These effects serve to increase perfusion of both brain and heart. In resuscitation, epinephrine is given to improve cerebral and cardiac blood flow. It is administered only after the infant is properly ventilated, since oxygen has to enter the lungs to reach the coronary and cerebral vessels, and epinephrine in the absence of adequate oxygen may cause tissue damage, especially to the myocardium.

The preferred route of administration is intravenous (IV). However, if placing an IV line (usually into the umbilical vein) takes too much time, one can administer epinephrine through an endotracheal tube. The dose of tracheal epinephrine must be higher than the dose of IV epinephrine would be for the same infant. Increased heart rate should be seen within 1 minute of giving IV epinephrine; it may take much longer, and may not be as effective, if given intratracheally.

Fluids, given through an umbilical line, may be needed for volume expansion in cases where the infant has lost considerable blood during delivery. Common reasons for blood loss include placenta previa, loss of blood from damage to the umbilical cord, and blood from the infant being lost into a twin or into the mother's circulation. The infant may be in hypovolemic shock, with bradycardia and poor perfusion that does not respond to ventilation, compression, or epinephrine. The most convenient fluids for volume expansion are normal saline and Ringer's lactate. O-negative packed red blood cells may be given in cases of fetal anemia; ideally the donor blood should be crossmatched to the mother to limit problems with maternal antibodies, but non-crossmatched O-negative blood can be given in dire emergencies. Volume expanders should not be used unless the infant is known to have lost blood acutely.

TRAINING IN NEONATAL RESUSCITATION

As neonatal resuscitation has evolved, so have the methods of training its providers. A major change occurred in 2011 with the publication of the 6th edition of the "Textbook of Neonatal Resuscitation" (2). Prior to that time; most NRP courses followed a lecture-demonstration-practice-test format that had been in place since NRP began. Now, we leave most of the didactics to the students themselves -- students are required to take the examination, on line, before starting the practical segment of the course -- and, although we still expect near-perfection with individual skills, the main part of the course consists of one or more simulated resuscitations in which a group of students conduct the resuscitation under the instructor's gaze, and then are debriefed with the instructor.

This is a considerable change from the old teaching methods. Instructors, instead of giving feedback in small doses through the class, keep it until the end, and in the debriefing have the students discuss (as individuals, but also as a team) what they did well and what they could improve upon. Debriefing is also intended for use after real resuscitations, so that after every delivery they attend they can review how well they performed and thereby build as a team on their latest experience as well as on their training and prior experiences. It is somewhat more demanding for instructors, but it helps us as well: we now concentrate on how the team, as well as its individual members, works together, and we also learn from our students' performance.

REFERENCES

[1] Black RE, Cousens S, Johnson HL, Lawn JE, Rudan I, Bassani DG, et al. Global, regional, and national causes of child mortality in 2008: a systematic analysis. Lancet 2010;375(9730):1969-87.

[2] Kattwinkel J, ed. Textbook of neonatal resuscitation, 6th ed. Elk Grove Village, IL: American Academy of Pediatrics and American Heart Association, 2011.

In: Born into this World: Health Issues
Editors: D. E. Greydanus, A. N. Feinberg et al.

ISBN: 978-1-63321-667-9
© 2014 Nova Science Publishers, Inc.

Chapter 6

BORN PREMATURE: WHAT DOES IT MEAN?

I Leslie Rubin[*], *MD*

Department of Pediatrics, Morehouse School of Medicine and Innovative
Solutions for Disadvantage and Disability, Atlanta, Georgia,
United States of America

ABSTRACT

Prematurity is the term used when a newborn infant is delivered before
term and is often associated with a low birth weight, of less than 2,500
grams. The concerns in the immediate neonatal period are for survival,
while later concerns are about health, growth and development. Over the
past 50 years, there has been an increasing focus of attention, research
and resources on assuring the survival and long term outcome of infants
who are born premature. As a result of advances in knowledge and
technology, there has followed an increased likelihood for survival of
even the smallest of premature infants. The challenges related to
promoting survival are offset by the increasing likelihood of a
neurologically based disability that is directly related to the degree of
prematurity. In addition, families face significant stresses associated with
the dramatic clinical picture in the immediate neonatal period and the
emotional stress continues for some time and needs to be taken into

---

[*] Correspondence: I Leslie Rubin, MD, Research Associate Professor, Department of Pediatrics,
Morehouse School of Medicine and President, Innovative Solutions for Disadvantage and
Disability, 776 Windsor Parkway, Atlanta, GA 30342, United States. E-mail:
lrubi01@emory.edu.

consideration. For these reasons, infants born prematurely require close monitoring for their health, growth and development and also for attention to family stresses.

INTRODUCTION

Premature birth rates continue to rise in the United States despite research and clinical efforts designed toward their reduction. Rates rose from 9.4% to 12.3% between 1981 and 2003, with most recent data showing the incidence at 12.7% (1). Preterm birth refers to all deliveries less than 37 weeks gestation (1).

> Centers for Disease Control (CD) report: Each year, preterm birth affects nearly 500,000 babies—that's 1 of every 8 infants born in the United States. Preterm birth is the birth of an infant prior to 37 weeks of pregnancy. Preterm-related causes of death together accounted for 35% of all infant deaths in 2009, more than any other single cause. Preterm birth is also a leading cause of long-term neurological disabilities in children. Preterm birth costs the U.S. health care system more than $26 billion in 2005.
> http://www.cdc.gov/reproductivehealth/maternalinfanthealth/PretermBirth.htm

The gestational ages can be viewed as very preterm (< 32 weeks), moderately preterm (32-33 weeks), and late preterm births (34-36). Term births refer to deliveries that occur from 37-42 weeks, and post-term births refer to any delivery occurring after 42 weeks.

Prematurity is also considered using birth weight as an indicator: infants born weighing less than 2,500 grams are considered low birth weight (LBW), those weighing less than 1,500 grams are considered very low birth weight (VLBW) weighing less than 1,000grams are considered to be of Extremely Low birth weight (ELBW). Advances in technology in the management of the premature infants have resulted in an increased survival of infants who weigh as little as 750-800 grams and of extreme prematurity as low as 23-24 weeks.

However, the linear measures of time of gestation or birth weight are not completely predictive of the real vulnerability of either the premature infants or the risks for neonatal complications and long term outcome in terms of intellectual or developmental disabilities (IDD). Factors such as immaturity of the central nervous system (CNS), lungs, gastrointestinal tract, endocrine, metabolic and immune systems compromise and complicate the ability of premature infant to survive and to develop appropriately.

The vulnerability of the premature infant to environmental factors is therefore fraught with great risk and with significant long term implications. The management strategies of these vulnerable infants in the immediate newborn period require corresponding rigor coupled with delicacy in managing the multiple physiological needs and in preventing injury and complications. The last five decades of care of the premature newborn infant have seen major changes with significant progress in technology and management strategies. This has been accomplished through creative research and continuous evaluation and reevaluation of practices and outcomes. Ultimately, the goal of management of the vulnerable premature infant is to limit insults to organ systems, particularly the CNS, and to assure optimal health, growth and developmental trajectories for the infant and for the family.

OBSTETRIC CONSIDERATIONS

The obstetric community is particularly concerned with prematurity because of their responsibility in caring for the pregnant mother and assuring optimal outcomes of the pregnancy for the mother and baby. While historically the focus of obstetricians was to assure a safe birth to reduce the risk of birth traumas as the cause of cerebral palsy and other developmental disabilities, prematurity today, in the western world in general and in the US in particular, represents the single most significant cause of cerebral palsy and birth related problems. Furthermore, while the primary concern around prematurity focuses on the smallest and most vulnerable of premature infants who are born under 32 weeks gestation, concern is rising about the outcomes of infants who are born between 34-37 weeks gestation. This group of infants who were previously considered to be at very low risk for IDD are now recognized as having relatively greater risk than the full term infants of gestational age 37-40 weeks but, obviously, significantly less than the infants who are born at less than 34 weeks gestation. This group of infants is referred to as 'late preterm births'.

Spontaneous premature delivery occurs in about 75% of premature births as a result of unexplained preterm labor in about 60% or premature rupture of the membranes in about 40% of cases. Premature delivery may also be a result of problems with the pregnancy requiring urgent obstetric intervention. In these situations obstetric intervention is indicated for preeclampsia in about

40%, markers of fetal distress in 25%, poor fetal growth in 10% and 7% for both placental abruption and fetal death (2).

FACTORS PREDISPOSING TO PREMATURITY

Factors contributing to prematurity can be clear in some cases while in others the reasons are obscure. Although risk factors can be divided into maternal, placental or fetal, in reality it is not always easy to sort out because many factors are interrelated, particularly social factors such as low income and minority status where the factors may be cumulative, compounding and confounding (3). Risk factors associated with prematurity:

Social, personal and economic characteristics
- Low or high maternal age
- Low maternal income or socioeconomic status
- Being African American

Medical and pregnancy conditions
- Prior preterm birth
- Maternal illness e.g., hypertension or diabetes
- Maternal infection
- Anatomical problems with uterus or cervix
- Multiple births (twins, triplets, or more)

Behavioral
- Stress
- Tobacco and alcohol use
- Substance abuse
- Late or no prenatal care

Maternal age is an important factor with an ideal age for health in pregnancy being somewhere between 18 and 35 years of age. While many women who tend to be more educated, are delaying childbearing because of personal and career choices, younger, often teenage girls, who tend to be from low income, minority and underserved communities are becoming pregnant. Both of these groups are at higher risk for prematurity. For the more educated women who seek to become pregnant later in life, there is more likely to be increased difficulty in conceiving, requiring a variety of fertility strategies, some of which result in multiple births, increasing the risk of prematurity (2). Although this phenomenon is increasing in many countries, the numbers of women remain relatively small compared to the population of less educated, low income women who become pregnant at the younger end of the age spectrum. This phenomenon is universal with reports from many parts of the world with the same finding of an increase in prematurity associated with low socioeconomic status, low educational level and minority status (3-5).

Maternal health and well-being are crucial to a healthy pregnancy for a desired full term outcome. Maternal illnesses such as diabetes, autoimmune disorders or hypertension or infections can significantly complicate the pregnancy and result in premature births. It is, however, in the realm of maternal behavior patterns and socioeconomic status that most of the risks for premature birth are found.

Interestingly, the behavioral risk factors such as tobacco use and substance abuse are also more prevalent in this population group and further complicate and compound the situation increasing the risk of preterm deliveries. Furthermore, stress factors are significantly higher and are associated with limited access to appropriate medical or mental health services, resulting in limited, poor or no prenatal care, self-medication and other risk behaviors.

There are also mechanical factors such as cervical incompetence and placental factors that predispose to prematurity but they are much less common. Placental abnormalities and placental dysfunction, particularly predisposing to intrauterine growth retardation (IUGR) can compromise the health of the fetus and complicate the neonatal course and long term outcome. Placental malposition—such as placental previa—can predispose to premature deliveries as can congenital anomalies in the fetus and multiple births.

NEONATAL COMPLICATIONS

Overall, the immediate newborn period of a premature infant is dramatic and complex, requiring attention to respiratory management and adequate oxygenation, cardiovascular stability, adequate hydration and nutrition, temperature stability, urine production, skin integrity, and many other considerations at different levels. Generally, smaller infants are more delicate to manage and more vulnerable and fraught with many potential complications. Although the birth weight and gestational age correlate directly with severity and complexity of neonatal complications as well as short term and long term outcomes, it is important to consider individual variation as a vital factor in immediate management and in the long term outcome. For this reason, any prognostications for parents at the early stages and even at discharge from the neonatal intensive care unit (NICU) should be given with cautious optimism.

The greatest challenge to the survival of a premature newborn infant is the ability to breathe. The deficiency of surfactant in the premature newborn infant results in collapse of the alveoli at each breath causing the infant to be very tired very quickly. This process rapidly devolves into the respiratory distress syndrome (RDS) requiring oxygen and intubation and assisted ventilation. This takes its toll on the cardiovascular system with consequent fluctuations in blood pressure that can be dramatic and have significant impact, particularly in the brain of the infant under 30 weeks gestation where delicate capillary walls can readily rupture with dramatic changes in pressure and result in hemorrhages with consequent damage to the delicate brain.

Another major risk is the delicate fluid and electrolyte balance, which can also affect cardiovascular stability. Other complications include jaundice, which can result in deposition of bilirubin in the brain, retinopathy of prematurity (ROP), necrotizing enterocolotis (NEC), as well as other frequent complications such as sepsis, hematological problems and other organ systems complications that require prompt attention.

Infants can spend months in the NICU, where they receive care and attention to all their physiological needs, as well as respiratory support, nutritional support, cardiovascular support, gastrointestinal and renal monitoring, and biochemical and hematological management. More often than not for the most premature infants, the early days are very much a dramatic life-or-death struggle until they become more stable and are transferred to a relative step-down unit to gain weight and grow until they are ready to go home. The length of stay in the NICU is directly related to the gestational age of the infant; those who are relatively less premature will leave earlier while those who are more premature may stay months. Often, premature infants will stay as long as it takes to reach the month of the correct time of birth, so an infant of 32 weeks gestational age will stay approximately two months, whereas if the infant is born at 28 weeks gestation he might stay approximately three months.

Since the 1970's when Klaus and Kennel revolutionized neonatal care by including and involving mothers and fathers in the care of their infants (6), more often than not, parents will be actively engaged with their premature infants and become quite literate, learning medical terminology and playing a more active role in the management of their baby's care. This is positive, and parents should be encouraged because there will come a day when the infants needs to go home and then the parents will need to be ready to care for their infant at home without any nursing or medical support, which can be quite daunting.

After the infant recovers from the stressful, and sometimes rather stormy neonatal course, consideration for the long term management becomes the focus of concern with attention to the chronic medical conditions and the neurodevelopmental concerns. These include the possibilities of bronchopulmonary dysplasia (BPD) from the RDS, visual impairment from the ROP, short bowel syndrome from the NEC and apneas and bradycardias that require a monitor.

This protracted length of time spent in the NICU inevitably takes its toll on the family's resources – physical, emotional, social and economic. Then, when the infants do eventually go home, the family has to deal with the reality of taking care of an infant who had been in a sophisticated medical setting for months and now is in the family's home with comparatively very little in the way of medical and nursing supports. As the medical problems are resolved, families soon turn their attention to the developmental outcomes and the stresses that these also bring to bear on the family's resources.

NEUROPATHOLOGICAL CONSIDERATIONS

The human brain develops from a neural plate, then a neural tube, then through the process of folding and septation, creates the basic form that the brain will take. What is then important is the population of neurons that develops and the migratory process that places the functioning neurons neatly layered in the cortex. This migratory process is critical to the development of connections between the neurons that will constitute the pathways for messages between the various parts of the brain. The final stage in the process is myelination, the insulation of the axons with layers of the myelin sheath that serves to speed up the transmission of impulses from one place in the brain to another. Most of the macro and micro architectural organization takes place before 40 weeks gestation, which is before birth, while most of the myelination proves takes place after 40 weeks, which is after birth.

There is a growing awareness of a specific network of neuronal connections that develops around 30 weeks of gestation that represents higher order brain functioning that speeds up processes of thought and cognition. These networks have been called the "rich club" because they economize on

                    I Leslie Rubin

neural pathways that have been likened to highway travel compared to travel on side roads, carrying large amounts of information that is functionally valuable in an efficient manner. Apparently these "rich club" networks evolve and consolidate between 30-40 weeks gestation (7,8).

Recent research suggests that although the "rich club" architecture is in place by 30 weeks, the period of time between 30-40 weeks gestation involves refinement, sophistication and enhancement of the "rich club" network. Therefore, if the infant is born prematurely, the further development of the 'rich club' nexus is vulnerable to pathophysiological insults which results in an altered network architecture with consequent reduced network capacity which contributes to the high prevalence of cognitive problems in preterm infants (9).

Furthermore, there is also growing awareness of the role played by interneurons such as oligodendrocytes and astroglia at a micro-architectural level involved in brain processing and function. These cells too are vulnerable in the premature infant, particularly as they also undergo myelination which can be interrupted by hypoxic insults (10).

HYPOXIA

The vulnerability of the preterm brain to the external environment and all the pathophysiological and pathological changes that happen to the premature infant in extrauterine life, alters the architecture and function of the brain, thereby altering the functional outcome of the individual with respect to thought and cognitive processes. Hypoxia and hypoxic ischemic encephalopathy of the premature infant are the most common causes of brain injury and subsequent functional impairment. Major sites in the brain that are affected include the cerebral white matter, particularly the periventricular area where the lesions of periventricular leukomalacia (PVL) are found, as well as the subplate and migrating neurons, the thalamus, basal ganglia and to some extent the cerebral cortex. Each of these areas has specific consequences on brain function and thus on cognitive, motor and social processing. The reader is referred to an excellent review on the encephalopathy of prematurity for more detail and background on the vulnerability of the premature brain to hypoxic insults (11).

HEMORRHAGE

The most common hemorrhages that occur in the premature infant are those involving the periventricular area. They occur more commonly in the younger premature infants because of the relatively unsupported vascularity in that area. The hemorrhages range in severity and are graded 1-4 with the higher grades being associated with hydrocephalus and with grade 4 being associated with parenchymal hemorrhages as well. Interestingly, reports of cerebellar hemorrhage are emerging with long term follow up suggesting significant sequelae (12,13).

One more recent emerging avenue of research is in the exploration of genetic determinants of vulnerability to brain insults in the premature infant (14). If genetic research proceeds as it has to date, we should have new and valuable information within a short period of time that will further help guide our clinical practices and go a long way to prevent disruptions in brain architecture by the insults of prematurity and perhaps even go a long way to preventing prematurity and its consequences.

NEUROLOGICAL SEQUELAE

For many years after the establishment and institution of the NICUs, the long term follow up of infants who were born prematurely and experienced stays in the NICU, were examined with a view as to whether they had intellectual impairment as documented by 2 standard deviations below the mean, or had clinical characteristics of cerebral palsy (CP) (15). If they did not fulfill those criteria, they were considered free of consequences. Over the course of time, however, we have become more sensitive and sophisticated in our evaluations of outcomes. Given the cumulative body of evidence, we are now looking at the complexity and intricacy of long term outcomes that include the family situation and the fact that many of the infants will now be in their mature adult years. We are also more closely examining many of the associated factors in the genesis of prematurity, practices in the NICU and the social and economic environments in which all this takes place.

                    I Leslie Rubin

MOTOR DISORDERS OF CEREBRAL PALSY

The association between birth related difficulties and motor disorders traces back to the 19th Century when William John Little (1810-1894) first reported to his colleagues at the Royal Society of Obstetricians in London and wrote his seminal article entitled: On the influence of abnormal parturition, difficult labor, premature birth and asphyxia neonatorum on mental and physical conditions of the child, especially in relation to deformities (16). Since that time, CP has been considered as a disorder of movement and posture as a result of a fixed insult to the developing brain before, during or soon after birth. Over the ensuing century and half in the western world, the perinatal causes of CP were related to birth trauma and birth asphyxia in term infants. Today, however, the etiological factors are related to prematurity and the complications of being born premature. This is not universal as there continue to be disparities around the world and in many other countries, particularly in parts of Africa and parts of Asia, the problems related to birth trauma and birth asphyxia for term infants persists.

The prevalence of CP is directly related to the birth weight and gestational age of the infant. A study in metropolitan Atlanta (17) found that the prevalence of CP was

- 59.5 per 1,000 live births among children born weighing less than 1,500 grams
- 6.2 per 1,000 live births among children born weighing 1,500 to 2,499 grams
- 1.1 per 1,000 for children born weighing 2,500 grams or more

In data from Sweden (18), the prevalence of CP was:

- 43.7 per 1,000 live births for children born at 28 to 31 weeks gestation
- 6.1 per 1,000 live births among children born at 32 to 36 weeks gestation
- 1.4 per 1,000 live births for children born at 37 or more weeks gestation

INTELLECTUAL AND DEVELOPMENTAL DISABILITIES (IDD)

It is well established that infants who are born prematurely are more likely to have learning and cognitive difficulties. Wilson-Costello and colleagues conducted a review of outcomes of infants from the early 1980s to the early 2000s, which revealed improved survival and improved overall outcome of extremely low birth weight infants. They cited a number of perinatal and neonatal factors that they felt were responsible for the improvement such as increased use of antenatal steroid, cesarean section delivery, decreased sepsis, decreased severe cranial ultrasound abnormalities, and postnatal steroid use despite no change in the rate of chronic lung disease (19).

Additionally a review of changes over two decades by Bode and colleagues (20) in Syracuse, New York reported a significant increase in live births at less than 30 weeks' gestational age, with a greater percentage of these neonates surviving without severe neurodevelopmental impairment at 24 months. On the other hand, a survey done in London, England looking at the short term outcomes of infants born between 22 to 26 weeks' gestation during 2006, compared the outcomes for babies born between 22 to 25 weeks' gestation since 1995, showed that while the survival of the infants increase, the pattern of major neonatal morbidity and the proportion of survivors affected was unchanged. This may well relate to the degree of prematurity in this study but none-the-less is an important consideration in reviewing practices and outcomes (21).

The constant review and scrutiny of outcomes related to NICU practices has clearly had substantial benefits both in terms of survival and in terms of improved outcome. We can only continue to examine and reexamine and revise our practices towards optimal outcomes for all.

ADHD AND AUTISM

We have come a long way since the early 1980s when we were looking at whether a child had the motor features of cerebral palsy or an intellectual disability to determine the consequences of prematurity, towards now examining other potential consequences. Along these lines we have come to appreciate that prematurity is indeed associated with an increased risk for attention deficit/hyperactivity disorder (ADHD), autism, and other behavior challenges as well (22-26). The data on the increase in likelihood of autism occurring in association with prematurity has been some time in coming but is emerging in a significant way. In 2008, Limperopoulos and colleagues reported on the finding of a greater than expected number of premature infants who scored positive on the "Modified checklist for autism in toddlers" (MCHAT); who had other findings on the Vineland and Child Behavior Checklist that were consistent with a diagnosis of Autism; and, whose magnetic resonance imaging (MRI) findings were also supportive of the diagnosis. They advised that early screening for signs of autism was warranted for premature infants, and if the screening is positive, they should obviously be followed with definitive autism testing and referral for appropriate services (27). This group has since reported on the rather strong association of cerebellar hemorrhage with adverse neurodevelopmental outcomes including a significant increase in autism (12).

LATE PRETERM BIRTHS

Late preterm births are those that take place between 34-37 weeks gestation. Late preterm newborns are the fastest growing subset of neonates, accounting for approximately 74% of all preterm births and about 8% of total births. While not considered technically premature, they have an increased risk for medical complications such as temperature instability, experience respiratory distress, become clinically jaundiced or need intravenous infusions. In addition to the immediate neonatal challenges there is a growing concern that this group of infants may have subtle neurodevelopmental consequences such as learning disabilities, behavior problems and, possibly, ADHD (2).

ADULT OUTCOMES

We have been following graduates of the NICUs for almost five decades, so we are able to look back and see how they are doing as adults. Their status depends significantly on the degree of prematurity, the degree of the insult to the developing brain, the resources within the family and community to meet the developmental and educational needs of the child, and the support that the child has in growing up and approaching life as an adult. A review by Hack and her colleagues in Cleveland strikes a rather positive note in recognizing that, while there are some difficulties, her group did not find serious antisocial behaviors (28).

SOCIAL DETERMINANTS

There is ample evidence from around the world that there are significant disparities in the rate of prematurity and in the outcomes of prematurity (3-5).

Even from early studies on the outcomes of premature infants graduating from the NICUs, there was a growing recognition that infants who grew up in homes where there were books and where parents were nurturing and talked to their infants the infants performed better on standardized tests than their counterparts who did not have those enriching experiences (15). At times, the variable was father's occupations, at times mother's education, and at times SES; however, overall the findings consistently suggested that infants born into circumstances of social and economic disadvantage did not fare as well on a variety of measures of functional outcome, from psychological test scores, to academic achievement, to later successes in life.

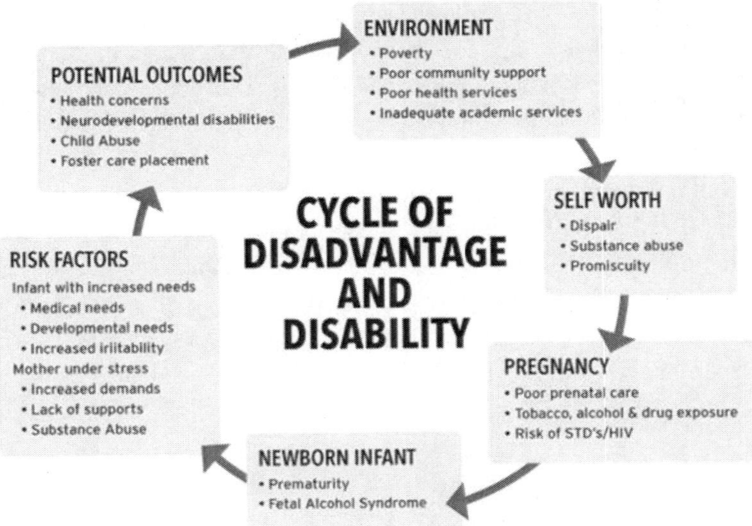

Figure 1. Cycle of disadvantage and disability.

The increased rate of prematurity among low income, minority populations is further compromised by the less than optimal social and educational environment which extends into the educational setting and future options and opportunities. This results in a closed system that can be viewed as a cycle of social and economic disadvantage and cognitive, educational and social disabilities (see figure 1)

Our challenge is to find a way to break the cycle at any point, during pregnancy, at delivery, in the NICU, at discharge from the NICU, at follow up visits, in early intervention programs at schools and, importantly, creating hope and a future for the children as they approach the threshold of maturity and become ready to start families of their own. (see chapter on Environmental Health Disparities)

COSTS OF CARE

The costs of an NICU stay vary from hospital to hospital and also with type of insurance coverage, as well as with the acuity and complexity of the needs of the premature infant. It follows that the more premature the infant, the more complex will be the clinical picture and the greater the cost of providing care. Moreover, the lower the gestational age of the premature infant the longer the infant will stay in the NICU and the greater will be the cumulative cost. The rough estimate is that it can cost between $1,000-$5,000 a day and that the average costs are estimated to be around $50,000, but can be as much as $500,000 in total for the youngest and most vulnerable of the premature infants (2,29).

In contrast, the average cost of early intervention for surviving premature infants in less than $1,000 but can go up to more than $5,000 for the most premature infants (30). Thus the full cost of early intervention services for each infant is roughly equivalent to the cost of one day's stay in the NICU.

This has led to the argument that it is better to prevent prematurity and invest more in early intervention and education of the graduates of the NICUs (31).

PERSONAL REFLECTIONS

The author had the opportunity and privilege to spend a year from 1976-1977 in the neonatal department of Marshall Klaus and Avroy Fanaroff at Rainbow Babies and Children's Hospital and Case Western Reserve University in

Cleveland, Ohio and reflected on the experience at that time. This is interesting in light of the progress that has taken place since then.

The atmosphere in the newborn nurseries and especially the neonatal intensive care units was abuzz with the spirit of learning new things every day, of studying challenging questions and of trying to make sure that every baby, no matter how premature or how small, would survive the challenges of breathing air, of requiring adequate nutrition to grow and develop normally, and of being able to tolerate the environmental vicissitudes of extra uterine life.

At this time, one could appreciate four major areas in which emerging knowledge and understanding would change the landscape of clinical pediatrics and of our society dramatically:

- The clinical and academic rigor in trying to understand the physiology and pathophysiology of the premature infants and what techniques and technologies could help to assure their healthy survival.
- The emerging technology of neuroimaging beginning with the Computerized Topographic (CT) Scans of the head and brain, and expanding to with use of Ultrasound and Magnetic Resonance Imaging (MRI) of the brain.
- The increasing appreciation of the fact that even if the infants could survive the neonatal period with all its stresses and insults, there was a likelihood that there would be physiological, medical, functional and social consequences.
- There was a critical need to include and involve parents, especially mothers, in the entire process. At the time, it was felt that this would assure that there was a positive relationship between the mother and infant – captured in the term of those days "Mother-Infant Bonding" – which would improve the likelihood of health and well-being for the infants and their families.

CONCLUSION

In the past five decades we have seen significant advances in management of pregnancy and delivery to the point that we can anticipate a successful outcome of any one pregnancy. Technological and scientific advances have also resulted in quantum leaps in our understanding of the physiology and pathophysiology of organ systems, particularly of the brain. Unfortunately, the rate of prematurity is high, and appears to be climbing, so that many more infants are being born prematurely today than before. But with advances in management of pregnancies and neonatal care, even the smallest infants born have a chance for survival into childhood and adulthood with varying degrees of success and difficulty.

What remains is the challenge of health disparity in the risk for prematurity and the risk for an adverse outcome for the children who live in low income, underserved and minority communities. It is tantalizing to contemplate that prematurity and its functional, social and financial implications can be prevented, thus saving much emotional, physical and financial resources to invest in the future of children and our society.

It is ironic that the daily cost for a preterm infant is estimated to be equivalent to the total cost of early intervention services for that infant, and leads us to ask questions about the cost of prevention and potential benefit to all. Moreover, if we could, in some way, redistribute that resources towards prevention of preterm deliveries among the most high risk and vulnerable women and invest some of it in early education with sustained quality education as we look to the future, we can make a substantial difference in outcomes of pregnancy, outcomes of premature births, and outcomes of good education, thus breaking the cycle (see figure 1) and benefitting all society.

ACKNOWLEDGMENTS

This paper is an adapted and revised version of an earlier publication: Rubin IL.

Prematurity and its consequences. In: Rubin IL, Merrick J, Greydanus DE, Patel DR, eds. Rubin and Crocker 3rd edition: Health care for people with intellectual and developmental disabilities across the lifespan. Dordrecht: Springer, 2014.

REFERENCES

[1]   Martin JA, Kung HC, Mathews TJ, Hoyert DL, Strobino DM, Guyer B, et al. Annual summary of vital statistics: 2006. Pediatrics 2008;121(4):788–801.

[2]   Loftin RW, Habli M, DeFranco EA. Late preterm birth. Rev Obstet Gynecol 2010;3:10-9.

[3]   Kramer MR, Hogue CR. What causes racial disparities in very preterm birth? A biosocial perspective. Epidemiol Rev 2009;31:84-98.

[4]   Donoghue D, Lincoln D, Morgan G, Beard J. Influences on the degree of preterm birth in New South Wales. Aust NZ J Public Health 2013;37:562-7.

[5]   Morgen CS, Bjørk C, Andersen PK, Mortensen LH, Andersen A-MN. Socioeconomic position and the risk of preterm birth. A study within the Danish National Birth Cohort. Int J Epidemiol 2008;37:1109-20.

[6]   Kennell JH, Klaus MH. Bonding: Recent observations that alter perinatal care. Pediatr Rev 1998;19:4-12.

[7]   Whalley K. Neuronal networks: In the rich club. Nature Rev Neurosci 2012;3:13.

[8]   van den Heuvel MP, Kersbergen KJ, de Reus MA, Keunen K, Kahn RS, Groenendaal F, et al. The neonatal connectome during preterm brain development. Cerebral Cortex 2014 May 15. doi:10.1093/cercor/bhu095

[9]   Balla G, Aljabara P, Zebaria S, Tusora N, Arichia T, Merchanta N, et al. Rich-club organization of the newborn human brain. PNAS 2014;111:7456-61.

[10]   Salmaso N, Jablonska B, Scafidi J, Vaccarin FM, Gallo V. Neurobiology of premature brain injury Nature Neuroscience 2014;17:341-6.

[11]   Volpe JJ. The encephalopathy of prematurity. Brain injury and impaired brain development inextricably intertwined. Semin Pediatr Neurol 2009;16:167-78.

[12]   Limperopoulos C, Bassan H, Gauvreau K, Robertson RL Jr, Sullivan NR, Benson CB, et al. Does cerebellar injury in premature infants contribute to the high prevalence of long-term cognitive, learning, and behavioral disability in survivors? Pediatrics 2007;120:584-93.

[13]   Limperopoulos C, Chilingaryan G, Sullivan N, Guizard N, Robertson RL, et al. Injury to the premature cerebellum: Outcome is related to remote cortical development. Cerebral Cortex 2012;24(3):728-36.

[14]   Boardman JP, Walley A, Ball G, Takousis P, Krishnan ML, Hughes-Carre L, et al. Common genetic variants and risk of brain injury after preterm birth. Pediatrics 2014;133;2013-30.

[15]   Wilson-Costello D, Hack M Follow-up for high-risk neonates. In: Martin RJ, Fanaroff AA, Walsh MC, eds. Fanaroff and Martin's neonatal-perinatal medicine: Diseases of the fetus and infant, 9th ed. St Louis, MO: Elsevier, 2011:1037-48.

[16]   Little WJ. On the influence of abnormal parturition, difficult labor, premature birth and asphyxia neonatorum on mental and physical conditions of the child, especially in relation to deformities. Trans Obstet Soc Lond 1862;3:293-344.

[17]   Winter S, Autry A, Boyle C, Yeargin-Allsopp M. Trends in the prevalence of cerebral palsy in a population-based study. Pediatrics 2002;110:1220-5.

[18]   Pakula AT, Van Naarden Braun K, Yeargin-Allsopp M. Cerebral palsy: Classification and epidemiology. In: Michaud LJ, ed. Cerebral palsy. Philadelphia, PA: WB Saunders, 2009:437.

[19]   Wilson-Costello D, Friedman H, Minich N, Siner B, Taylor G, Schluchter M, Hack M. Improved neurodevelopmental outcomes for extremely low birth weight infants in 2000-2002. Pediatrics 2007;119:37-45.

                                    I Leslie Rubin

[20]   Bode MM, D'Eugenio DB, Forsyth N, Coleman J, Gross CR, Gross SJ Outcome of extreme prematurity: A prospective comparison of 2 regional cohorts born 20 Years apart. Pediatrics 2009;124:866-74.

[21]   Costeloe KL, Hennessy EM, Haider S, Stacey F, Marlow N, Draper ES, Short term outcomes after extreme preterm birth in England: comparison of two birth cohorts in 1995 and 2006 (the EPICure studies). BMJ 2012;345:e7976.

[22]   Lou HC. Etiology and pathogenesis of attention-deficit hyperactivity disorder (ADHD): Significance of prematurity and perinatal hypoxic-haemodynamic encephalopathy. Acta Paediatr 1996;85:1266-71.

[23]   Bhutta AT, Cleves MA, Casey PH, Cradock MM, Anand KJS. Cognitive and behavioral outcomes of school-aged children who were born preterm: A meta-analysis. JAMA 2002;288(6):728-37.

[24]   Msall ME, Park JJ. The spectrum of behavioral outcomes after extreme prematurity: regulatory, attention, social, and adaptive dimensions. Semin Perinatol 2008;32(1):42-50.

[25]   Feldman R, Eidelman AI. Neonatal state organization, neuromaturation, mother-infant interaction, and cognitive development in small-for-gestational-age premature infants. Pediatrics 2006;118:e869-78.

[26]   Hack M, Taylor HG, Schluchter M, Andreias L, Drotar D, Klein N. Behavioral outcomes of extremely low birth weight children at age 8 years. J Dev Behav Pediatr 2009;30(2):122-30.

[27]   Limperopoulos C, Bassan H, Sullivan NR, Soul JS, Robertson Jr RL, Moore M, et al. Positive screening for autism in ex-preterm infants: Prevalence and risk factors. Pediatrics 2008;121(4);758-65.

[28]   Hack M, Flannery DJ, Schluchter M, Cartar L, Borawski E, Klein N. Outcomes in young adulthood for very-low-birth-weight infants. N Engl J Med 2002;346:149-57.

[29]   St John EB, Nelson KG, Cliver SP, Bishnoi RR, Goldenberg RL. Cost of neonatal care according to gestational age at birth and survival status. Am J Obstet Gynecol 2000;182:170-5.

[30]   Clements KM, Barfield WD, Ayadi MF, Wilber N. Preterm birth-associated cost of early intervention services: an analysis by gestational age. Pediatrics 2007;119(4):e866-74.

[31]   Muraskas J, Parsi K. The cost of saving the tiniest lives: NICUs versus prevention. Virtual Mentor 2008;10(10):655-8.

In: Born into this World: Health Issues   ISBN: 978-1-63321-667-9
Editors: D. E. Greydanus, A. N. Feinberg et al.   © 2014 Nova Science Publishers, Inc.

Chapter 7

CIRCUMCISION

Julian Wan, MD[*]

Department of Urology, University of Michigan Medical Center,
Ann Arbor, Michigan, United States of America

In this review we discuss circumcision, its indications (anatomic, socio-economic, and preventive). We then outline procedural techniques and review contraindications and complications. Finally we discuss alternatives to circumcision and present recent political issues regarding this subject.

Keywords: Circumcision, phimosis, paraphimosis, balanitis, GOMCO, Plastibell, neonatal circumcision

INTRODUCTION

Circumcision is among mankind's most common and oldest procedures. It is also historically one of the most controversial. The reasons for its performance range from religious rite, social habit and convention, medical therapy and prophylaxis. The latter categories include phimosis, paraphimosis, hygiene, and reducing the relative risk to urinary tract infections and sexually

---

[*] Correspondence: Professor Julian Wan, Department of Urology, University of Michigan Medical Center, 3875 Taubman Center, 1500 East Medical Center Drive, Ann Arbor, MI 48109, United States. E-mail: juliwan@umich.edu

transmitted diseases (STDs) including human immunodeficiency virus (HIV)
(1). Removal of the prepuce exposes the tip of the penis and changes the
microenvironment of the glans. The glanular epithelium undergoes metaplasia,
changing from a moist glabrous transitional and translucent tissue to a dry
tough squamous layer. Whether the risks and benefits justify this change
continues to be the subject of debate and discussion.

INDICATIONS FOR CIRCUMCISION

The non-religious and non-social indications for circumcision can be divided
into two groups. The first group applies to those older children who were not
circumcised at birth and who later encounter difficulties with the foreskin. The
second group includes those who have circumcision prior to developing any
problems in hopes of preventing or lessening risk of future difficulties; these
are largely the reasons given for neonatal circumcision. For children who were
not circumcised at birth, the indications mainly relate to difficulties with
retracting or repositioning the prepuce. Between the ages of 5 to 7 years old,
the foreskin in the typical boy can be retracted to expose the glans partially or
fully. If the foreskin does not fully retract earlier in life it should not be
regarded as an abnormality as it is a normal physiological form of phimosis.
After that age, continued difficulty with retracting the prepuce becomes a true
pathological phimosis. Circumcision is the most straightforward solution.
Alternatives include a dorsal slit procedure and application of steroid
ointments (2) which can in mild cases loosen up the foreskin sufficiently to
obviate any procedure. These are options often selected by families in whom a
desire not to appear circumcised is socially important. Other difficulties with
the foreskin, such as paraphimosis, balanoposthitis, and lesions on the prepuce
itself may also require circumcision (1).

INDICATION FOR CIRCUMCISION FOR RELIGIOUS RITE, SOCIO-ECONOMIC REASONS AND MEDICAL PROPHYLAXIS

The second group of indications for circumcision comprises those reasons
where the foreskin is not causing a direct problem. They include religious
rites, social reasons, and situations where circumcision may lessen the risk of
other problems later in life. The oldest indications for a circumcision are

related to religious rites. The two best known groups who perform circumcision are followers of the Jewish and Islamic faiths. In many ways the indications are the most straightforward. The family either chooses to follow the rite or not. It should be noted that all of the major religions who have circumcision as a rite make allowances for medical contraindications, which may endanger the child's health or life (1).

ECONOMICS

When compared to the cost of treating balanitis, paraphimosis, true phimosis and conditions such as penile cancer and HIV, the relatively small cost of a neonatal circumcision has been advanced as an argument to justify preemptive circumcision as long term cost-saving measure. Some insurance plans no longer cover routine neonatal circumcision. Might neonatal circumcision be cost effective in the long run?

In a Gedanken experiment (thought experiment) it is argued that it would be cost effective, even if only 10% of the children develop problems later in life, and would prevent a much greater expenditure in costs. As an example were neonatal circumcision to cost $125 and if 2 million were done each year, it would cost $250 million per year. An adult circumcision in this discussion was calculated to cost $2000 and if there were 200,000 done each year (10% of the 2 million), it would cost a total cost of $400 million.

While an interesting intellectual exercise, the conclusion of this argument clearly varies tremendously with the number of circumcisions and how costs are calculated. This argument also neglects the potential costs of any complications.

While not entirely convincing currently this type of analysis will become more important in light of how the evolving discussion of how health care is funded. If there is a national initiative at limiting future medical costs by preventive actions in childhood or infancy this will undoubtedly be an important part of that discussion (3).

PENIS CANCER PREVENTION

Penile cancer is a rare condition. The typical patient is elderly and is uncircumcised. Fewer than a dozen cases have been reported in patients who are circumcised. The prepuce is the second most common site of origin after the glans penis and there has been theorized links with hygiene and STD exposure. Circumcision is postulated in some studies to reduce the risk by removing a high risk region and by improving hygiene and lowering the risk to STDs. Critics note that there are no data control for hygiene and STD exposure and other factors such as smoking, sexual activity, and other medical conditions of the penis that may play important roles (1).

CERVICAL CANCER LINKS

Cervical cancer is the second most common cancer in women worldwide and 99% may be attributable to infection by oncogenic human papilloma virus (HPV) genotypes. Infection with HPV subtypes 16 and 18 is implicated in 70% of cases and has been strongly associated with an increased risk of developing cervical carcinoma in women. The inner prepuce has been implicated as a possible harbor for the virus. Studies comparing the HPV infection rates of women whose partners are circumcised or uncircumcised have shown a marked difference.

Among uncircumcised men, up to 20% will harbor HPV whereas only 5.5 % of circumcised men will have the virus. Would widespread circumcision, therefore, lead to a drop in the cervical cancer incidence? The relative low risk of the vaccine and the data showing benefits have reached the point that routine vaccination has now become recommended (4,5).

URINARY TRACT INFECTIONS

The foreskin has been implicated as possible site to harbor bacteria associated with urinary tract infections. Several studies have noted that young circumcised males rarely develop UTIs when compared to uncircumcised boys. Wiswell and Rocscelli's retrospective study from 1974 to 1983 in over 200,000 girls and 200,000 boys found that 0.57% of the girls developed UTIs (6). Of the boys, 0.11% of the circumcised boys developed UTI as compared to 1.12% of the uncircumcised boys. This work and that of others suggest the odds of a UTI if uncircumcised are about 12 times that of the circumcised. The retrospective nature of the study could not control for other major risk factors such as vesicoureteral reflux and uretero-pelvic junction obstruction.

SEXUALLY TRANSMITTED DISEASES

Circumcision has been long considered a method of reducing the risk of sexually transmitted disease. The absence of the foreskin eliminates another moist harbor for the often fragile STD pathogens. The transformation of the skin of the glans to a tough squamous epithelium may also make it more resistant to penetration and infection. Studies conducted in the past looked at this issue but often were confounded by factors such as overall hygiene, sexual habits, and frequency. Until recently there were no randomized studies with a defined control group.

Three recent papers looking at the risk of a specific STD, namely HIV, have provided the first evidence supporting this hypothesis. The South African "Orange Farm" study by Auvert et al. (7) of 2005 studied the effects of circumcision in 3,000 young men aged 18 to 24 years. All were sexually active and followed for a two year period of time. The subjects were randomized with half undergoing immediate circumcision and the other half at the end of the study. By 21 months there was clear difference in the infection rate with HIV with a greater than 2 to 1 infection rate difference. Criticisms of this study included the short follow up period and two more randomized studies were conducted.

The Kenyan study by Bailey and et al (8) in 2007 enrolled over 4,400 men with 2,800 completing the study (8). They were randomized with 1400 undergoing immediate circumcision and the other control half being circumcised at the end of the study. Within 24 months the control group had a new HIV positive rate of 4.2% as compared with the circumcised group rate of 2.1%. A third study by Gray et al (9) in 2007 conducted around the same time occurred in Uganda in a broader group of men with ages ranging from 15 to 49 years. Randomization formed a group of 2,400 men who underwent circumcision with a control group of 2,500. There was again a statistically significant difference at 24 months. Only 1.1% of the circumcision group became HIV positive whereas 2.6% of the control group became positive.

Together these studies show that circumcision can alter the risks of STD transmission in a statistically significant manner. There remains however the practical application of this finding. The circumcision did not prevent or eradicate HIV infection; it only lessened the risk in the short period of the study. Continued unprotected sexual activity would erode any advantage derived from the procedure over time. For this reason, while these are landmark papers in establishing the validity of the concept that altering the microenvironment of the glans penis can have a significant effect on the risk of infection by STDs, the practical benefits may be thwarted by personal behavior and habits.

CIRCUMCISION PROCEDURE, CONTRAINDICATIONS AND COMPLICATIONS

Circumcision is not a trivial procedure to be delegated to the inexperienced and unprepared. If done properly it is merely a short entry in a patient's medical history. However, when it is not approached in a careful manner the consequences can be devastating. For practitioners who plan on performing circumcision formal training is advisable. A period of time working with an experienced operator is strongly recommended.

There are two major techniques used for circumcision. For older infants and children, the typical method is the sleeve circumcision. After successful induction of general anesthesia the foreskin is retracted fully and any adhesions are taken down. A cuff of preputial skin about 0.7 to 1 cm from the corona of the glans is marked following the curve of the corona. A corresponding proximal circumferential line on the penile shaft is then marked off. An incision is made on these marks thereby isolating a cylinder of foreskin. This skin is removed and the edges are brought together using fine absorbable sutures. This method requires general anesthesia in children and infants but is advantageous in that it allows compensations for irregularities in shaft skin. The main disadvantage of this technique is its limitation to those who have formal surgical training and anesthesia requirement.

The other major technique is used almost exclusively for newborns and involves the use of a purpose built device to perform the circumcision. The two most common devices used in the US are the GOMCO™ clamp and the Plastibell™ system. Both of these techniques are usually performed under local anesthetic and produce a good cosmetic result with excellent hemostasis. The technique can be used successfully by non-surgeons who have received specific training. Hospitalists at our institutions have been successfully trained to do nearly all of the neonatal circumcisions.

There are four key points to remember when considering this technique. First, find a method which is agreeable, standardize it, and practice it. Experience will increase speed and facility. Second, be patient with hemostasis. Both the GOMCO™ and Plastibell™ have explicit instructions on the length of time the device should be applied for optimal hemostasis. In the

GOMCO the time is at least 5 minutes. Trying to save a few minutes by not waiting the recommended period of time is a foolish expediency.

Third, examine the patient carefully and become familiar with the normal variations in the appearance of the glans, urethral meatus, foreskin, and shaft. Normal variations such as megameatus, penile skin torsion and penoscrotal webbing should recognizable on sight and differentiated from anomalies which would defer the circumcision, especially hypospadias. Fourth, never use electrocautery when doing a neonatal circumcision, especially with the GOMCO clamp. Misuse of electrocautery by inexperienced operators have resulted in near and complete destruction of the phallus.

Due to the new research on STD and HIV there has been interest in developing similar devices for use in adults. This would allow non-surgically trained personnel to perform circumcision under local anesthetic. A variety of devices are being promoted but as of the time of this chapter none has yet become as established as the GOMCO™ or Plastibell™ (10).

CONTRAINDICATIONS TO CIRCUMCISION

The contraindications to circumcision resemble those of any elective procedure. Patients who have a known bleeding disorder such as hemophilia or von Willebrand's disease should be deferred. Those whose penis is less than 1 cm stretched length at birth or whose girth is less than 1 cm should be deferred. Urethral and glanular anomalies such as hypospadias, penoscrotal webbing, buried penis or marked chordee are contraindications. Finally if the baby is sick, the circumcision should be deferred until the baby is well.

COMPLICATIONS

The most important complication is failure to recognize hypospadias. Repair of hypospadias after the foreskin has been removed is more difficult. Necrosis of shaft skin and glans may occur if epinephrine is used when infiltrating a local block or if electrocautery is used injudiciously. As noted, never use electrocautery when performing neonatal circumcision involving the Plastibell™ or GOMCO™ devices. Always be sure that when using the Plastibell™ that the caregivers bring the baby back within one week to be sure the ring has fallen off. Left on too long the ring can deform the glans.

Laceration of the glans or amputation of the tip of the glans can occur if one of the older blind circumcision techniques is used. It is also seen as a complication of circumcision device such as the Mogen clamp. Immediate re-anastomosis of the glans is usually successful.

Bleeding can occur along the edge of the incised skin, from penetrating vessels on the shaft or from the frenulum. Direct pressure, suture ligature, and the very careful use of fine needle point electrocautery should be able to control nearly all cases. Be suspicious of bleeding disorders when infants and young children have intra-operative or post-operative bleeding problems.

Infections are rare and localized infections can be treated with topical or oral antibiotics with drainage. Systemic infections including Fournier's gangrene have been reported but fortunately are exceptionally rare. Aggressive therapy with parenteral antibiotics and debridement of necrotic tissue is needed. Separation of the circumcision seam can occur but usually resolves well. When it occurs within the first week of life, it usually heals spontaneously with excellent cosmesis. The treatment is usually copious amounts of antibiotic ointment on the tip and careful observation. Skin grafting and surgery are not advised. One reason for separation is that positioning the clamp without accounting for the coronal angulation may leave the ventral shaft skin remnant short and under tension. Redundant residual foreskin can occur when an insufficient or uneven amount of foreskin had been resected. Treatment is usually a revision circumcision.

Adhesions usually result from residual foreskin clinging to the glanular corona. These can be either peeled back or resected as part of a revision circumcision. Skin bridges or bands can occur when a narrow web of skin grows from the circumcision seam onto the glans. These create pockets of dead space into which smegma and other debris can accumulate. Treatment involves sharply taking down these bands flush against the glans and penile shaft. Penile torsion and chordee can occur if there is unevenness or twist in the shaft skin. The usual treatment is to take down the penile shaft skin and try to correct the imbalance.

Glanular division can occur during the vertical slitting of the foreskin. Taking down preputial adhesions prior to cutting and awareness of this complication are the key points in prevention. Treatment is primary repair and closure over a catheter if the urethra is involved. Inclusion cysts can occur when portions of the skin become buried during closure. This results in a buried space which over time fills with smegma and debris. Treatment is excision of the cyst and its lining.

Urethral injuries and urethrocutaneous fistula can occur when sutures used to control bleeding inadvertently catch the urethra. Treatment is primary closure. When the fistula is close to the glans tip, it is preferable to split the glans down to the fistula and recreate the distal urethra using a hypospadias technique. Urinary retention can occur due to secondary phimosis or overly tight dressing. Suture tracks occur when the paths of the dissolving sutures do not collapse but become keratinized tunnels. The tracks fill with lint and other debris giving the appearance of small dark spots and streaks. Treatment is unroofing these tracks sharply. To prevent the development of these tracks, inverted buried closure has been advocated. Meatal stenosis has been identified as a long term possible complication of neonatal circumcision. Up to 7% of circumcised neonates later developed meatal stenosis (11).

ALTERNATIVES TO CIRCUMCISION

When a child has an indication for a circumcision there are a few alternative treatments which can be considered should the family have a strong personal reason for not wanting the child to be circumcised. Topical corticosteroid creams such as betamethasone have been shown to have benefit in some children (2). They are theorized to have two possible mechanisms: anti-inflammatory as well as immunosuppressive effect and skin thinning. Corticosteroids stimulate the production of lipocortin that in turn suppresses phospholipase A2, which releases arachidonic acid from phospholipids. Part of the anti-inflammatory effect is to reduce Type I and III collagen synthesis in many cells including fibroblasts. Second there is a skin thinning effect. Steroids inhibit dermal synthesis of glycosaminoglycans by fibroblasts resulting in a loss of the ground substance thereby reducing the extracellular matrix and have an active role in inhibiting collagen synthesis in the epidermis.

For patients whose phimosis is recalcitrant to treatment with corticosteroids, an alternative procedure is a dorsal slit. Rather than removing the foreskin, a vertical cut is made into the foreskin along the dorsal side. This cut extends the circumference of the foreskin opening thereby making it easier to retract. The foreskin is left intact but the procedure requires local or general anesthesia and cosmetically the result may be an odd-appearing ventral apron.

HEALTH POLITICS

The evolution of the understanding about the effects of circumcision has run parallel with changes in official health policy and their political ramifications. The African circumcision studies led to the issuance of statement from the World Health Organization in 2007 which officially recognized that male circumcision "should be part of a comprehensive HIV prevention package". The American Academy of Pediatrics in 2012 changed their official position to reflect these changes: "evaluation of current evidence indicates that the health benefits of newborn males outweigh the risks and that the procedure's benefits justify access to this procedure for families who choose it" (1). The American College of Obstetrics and Gynecology whose members still perform up to half of the neonatal circumcisions in some areas endorsed this position as well. While not a sweeping endorsement it represents a marked change from their earlier position which previously held that "existing scientific evidence demonstrates potential medical benefits of newborn male circumcision; however, these data are not sufficient to recommend routine neonatal circumcision."

During this time efforts worldwide to curtail the practice of female circumcision which is essentially a clitorectomy drew interest in forming a parallel discussion about male neonatal circumcision. If female circumcision is to be banned, the argument was advanced to also include male neonatal circumcision. Bills under the heading of "male genital mutilation" has been submitted for consideration by the US House of Representatives and Senate but has not progressed any further. Local efforts on a municipal level have also been submitted but have not been enacted in the US.

In Europe, the issue arose when a local appellate court in Cologne, Germany citing the Human Rights Provision of the Basic Law section of the German legal code ruled that religious circumcision of male children equated bodily injury and is a criminal offense under its jurisdiction. Jewish, Islamic and ethnic groups (particularly the sizable Turkish minority) protested that this was an attack on religious freedom because circumcision was an integral religious ritual.

In July 2012 a unique alliance of these groups issued a joint statement denouncing this ruling and asked relief from the German courts and the European Parliament. The major German political parties from the political right, center, and left formed a second unique alliance and drafted a specific law stipulating that male circumcisions be allowed so long as they can be performed without pain and in accordance with best medical practice. The law was passed and enacted as part of German Civil Code effective Dec. 28, 2012.

This was not the final word on the subject. Several of the prominent professional medical bodies came out formally against neonatal circumcision. The German Academy for Pediatric and Adolescent Medicine (Deutsche Akademie für- Kinder und Jugend medizin e.V., DAKJ), The German Association for Pediatric Surgery (Deutsche Gesellschaft für Kinderchirurgie, DGKCH), and the Professional Association of Pediatric and Adolescent Physicians (Berufsverband der Kinder- und Jugendärzte) issued a statement firmly opposing non-medically indicated routine infant circumcision.

The current situation is still in flux. Further complicating the discussion is the medical-legal liability issue. Some have advanced the notion that since HIV transmission is lowered among the circumcised, might there be liability issues by NOT offering neonatal circumcision to parents? Clearly this is a topic which remains controversial and will continue be so for the foreseeable future (12-16).

CONCLUSION

In summary, circumcision is an ancient yet common procedure. It is performed for social, religious, and medical reasons inspiring much research, debate and discussion. Though simple and quick to perform, circumcision requires a serious approach.

REFERENCES

[1]   Task Force on Circumcision. Circumcision policy statement. Pediatrics 2012;130(3):e756-85.

[2]   Ashfield JE, Nickel KR, Siemens Dr, MacNeily AE, Nickel JC. Treatment of phimosis with topical steroids in 194 children. J Urol 2003;169(3):1106-8.

[3]   Cadman D, Gafni A, Mcnamee J. Newborn circumcision: an economic perspective. Can Med Assoc J 1984;131:1353-5.

[4]   Castellsague X, Bosch FX, Munoz N, Meijer CJLM, Shah KV, de Sanjose S, et al. Male circumcision, penile human papillomavirus infection, and cervical cancer in female partners. N Engl J Med 2002; 346(15):1105-12.

[5]   The Advisory Committee on Immunization Practices of the Centers for Disease Control and Prevention. HPV vaccine recommendations. Pediatrics 2012;129(3):602-5.

[6]   Wiswell TE and Roscelli JD. Corroborative evidence for the decreased incidence of urinary tract infections in circumcised male infants. Pediatrics 1986;78(1):96-9.

[7]   Auvert B, Taljaard D, Lagarde E, Sobngwi-Tambekou J, Sitta R, Puren A. Randomized,controlled intervention trial of male circumcision for reduction of HIV infection risk:the ANRS 1265 Trial. PLoS Med 2005; 2:e298-304.

[8]   Bailey RC, Moses S, Parker CB, Agot K, Maclean I, Krieger JN, et al. Male circumcision for HIV prevention in young men in Kisumu, Kenya: a randomised controlled trial. Lancet 2007;369(9562):643–56.

[9]   Gray RH, Kigozi G, Serwadda D, Makumbi F, Watya S, Nalugoda F, et al. Male circumcision for HIV prevention in men in Rakai, Uganda: a randomised trial. Lancet 2007;369(9562):657–66.

[10]   Wan J. GOMCO Circumcision clamp: An enduring and unexpected success. Urol 2002;59:790-94.

[11]   Gee WF, Ansell JAS. Neonatal circumcision: A ten-year overview: with comparison of the Gomco Clamp and the Plastibell Device. Pediatrics 1976;58:824-7.

[12]   Der Bundestag hat am Donnerstag, 19. Juli 2012, in einer Sondersitzung folgende Beschlüsse gefasst: URL: http://www.bundestag.de/dokumente/textarchiv/2012/ 39861243_kw29_angenommen_abgelehnt/index.html [German]

[13]   Deutsche Akademie für Kinder- und Jegenmedizin. Stellungnahme zur Beschneidung von minderjahrigen Jungen Kommission für ethische Fragen der DAKJ. URL: http://www.dgkic.de/index.php/presse/189-pressemitteilung-juli-2012 [German]

[14]   CNN.com Law Center: A proposed bill to ban male circumcision. URL: http://www.cnn.com/2005/LAW/04/08/colb.circumcision/

[15]   San Francisco Circumcision ban: An attack on religious freedom. TIME 2011 Jun13. URL: http://content.time.com/time/nation/article/0,8599,2077240,00.html

[16]   Jewish groups condemn court's definition of circumcision as grievous bodily harm. Telegraph 2012 Jun 27 2012.

In: Born into this World: Health Issues
Editors: D. E. Greydanus, A. N. Feinberg et al.
ISBN: 978-1-63321-667-9
© 2014 Nova Science Publishers, Inc.

Chapter 8

ENVIRONMENT AND BIRTH WEIGHT

Rebecca Ouyang, BA[*]

Nicholas School of the Environment, Duke University, NC, US

A growing body of research has broadened the study of the relationship between the built environment and health from individual housing conditions to include the larger neighborhood environment and its subsequent effects on residents' health outcomes. Research has connected measures of neighborhood quality to changes in health outcomes for residents, yet little research has been done to develop measures that capture and quantify the physical features of the neighborhood's man-made surroundings, also known as the built environment. This paper investigates the current literature detailing the relationship between the built environment and low birth weight and suggests potential interventions. Interventions developed at the county, neighborhood, and individual levels could aid community leaders and policymakers in breaking the cycle of low birth weight.

INTRODUCTION

Public health researchers have long recognized the link between housing and health. Much of the current research available linking health outcomes to

---

[*] Correspondence: Rebecca Ouyang, Duke University, Nicholas School of the Environment, Children's Environmental Health Initiative, Box 90328, Durham, NC 27708. E-mail: rebecca.ouyang@gmail.com

housing focuses on the direct physical pathways of the housing conditions such as damp, cold, mold, heat, or homelessness (1-3). Recent research has begun to broaden the study to the larger neighborhood environment and its subsequent effects on residents' health outcomes (4,5). While many studies have developed measures for neighborhood quality, little objective observational research has been conducted on one of the most important features of neighborhood conditions, the neighborhood's built environment.

The built environment is defined as the man-made environment, which takes into account physical conditions of the home, in addition to other buildings, spaces and products that are created or modified by people, including schools, workplaces, parks/recreations areas, business areas and roads (6). The structure of the built environment shapes indoor and outdoor physical environments as well as social environments and consequently, health and quality of life.

This paper investigates the association between a poor built environment and adverse birth outcomes, as indicated by low birth weight. Recent research has suggested that perceptions of neighborhood physical disorder, ranging from litter to run-down buildings, can exert a sense of fear and anxiety in residents of disadvantaged neighborhoods (7,8). Residents may perceive signs of physical disorder, such as vandalism or graffiti, as indicators of crime and a lack of mutual respect in the community, raising mistrust and fear (9). As a result of heightened stress in pregnant mothers, it is possible that a poor built environment can perpetuate a cycle of disadvantage and disability (see figure 1). The cycle of disadvantage and disability depicts how a poor environment can exert negative health outcomes on pregnant mothers, resulting in poor birth outcomes for their infants. Negative birth outcomes can result in psychological and developmental problems in children, affecting their education and job opportunities in the future. A lack of opportunities may then trap them in neighborhoods with inadequate health and academic services, perpetuating the cycle.

A poor built environment may act as a stressor for pregnant mothers leading them to turn to harmful behaviors such as substance abuse that can result in low birth weight children (10). A low birth weight child faces increased health risks that may impact their development during childhood and manifest in health outcomes that persist into adulthood. For example, infants that are born underweight face a higher risk of dying during their early months and years (11). Low birth weight children are more likely to experience combinations of various behavioral, health and neuropsychological problems, which can carry long-term consequences (12). These children often score significantly lower on intelligence tests than do children of normal birth weight, affecting their performance in school as children, and job opportunities and performance in adulthood (13,14).

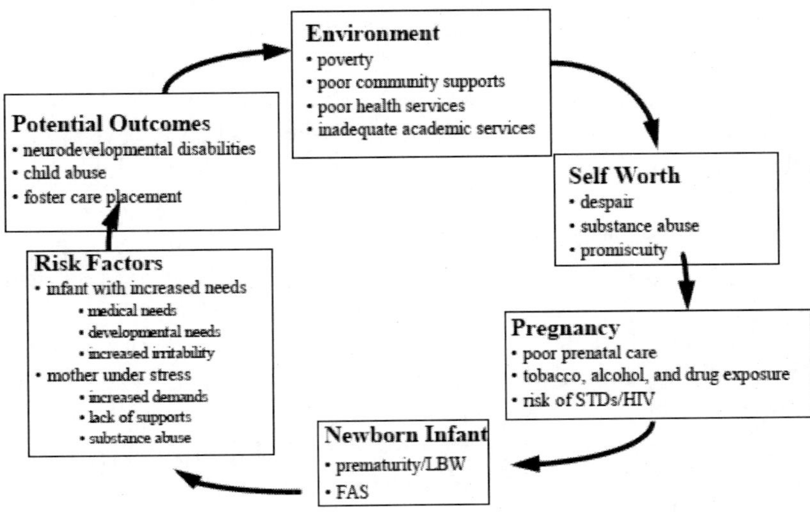

Figure 1. Cycle of disadvantage and disability.

While there has been some research elucidating the broader role of the neighborhood and its impact on birth outcomes, the traditional measures used to assess neighborhood quality are based on subjective individual perceptions or Census data that describes the socioeconomic demographics of the neighborhood's residents. These measures only reflect the aggregation of characteristics of individual residents but to not address the physical disorder (e.g., broken windows, peeling paint) present in the neighborhood. Therefore, there is a need for studies that employ objective observational ratings across multiple ecological contexts to evaluate physical neighborhood conditions. An understanding of the role that the neighborhood plays in its effect on maternal health and pregnancy outcomes could aid public health and housing policymakers in designing policies that would reduce the incidence of low birth weight.

This paper reviews the current literature on the built environment and its effects on health outcomes, specifically in relation to low birth weight. A review of the literature that examines the relationship between the built environment and birth weight will help elucidate the pathways between the two and highlight research gaps that still need to be explored and interventions that would help to reduce the low birth weight rate among women of lower socio-economic status.

SEARCH AND FINDINGS

A preliminary search on the Duke University Libraries article database was first conducted using the resources of Academic OneFile, Academic Search Premier, Business Source Complete, JSTOR, ProQuest, Project Muse and Web of Science.

The following terms were used in various combinations with one another for the preliminary search: built environment, neighborhood health, neighborhood quality, maternal stress, and low birth weight. Following this basic preliminary search, a selection process identified relevant articles. Additional articles were included by examining works cited by the authors of these articles.

Four main themes emerged from the current literature: 1) pathways between the built environment and health outcomes, (2) maternal stress and birth weight, (3) social capital as a mediating factor of stress, and (4) traditional measures of neighborhood quality. Each of these themes is discussed in detail below.

Pathways between the built environment and health outcomes

The built environment comprises a wide range of factors that include both the indoor and outdoor environment along with physical structures, roads, and sidewalks. As a result, many theories about the relationship between the built environment and health have evolved to explain how neighborhoods can affect health. Shaw (3) described a 2x2 matrix with the multiple combinations of the direct and indirect, and material and social ways that this happens. She describes not only the direct physical factors as the material effects of housing on health like damp, cold, mold, and heat that can compromise one's immune system, but also indirect physical factors that may serve as indicators for socioeconomic status in relation to income and wealth. Socioeconomic status in turn, then determines the availability of services and facilities. The social factors that directly affect health consider the effect of poor housing on mental health and the feeling of "home", and social status. Indirect social factors examine culture in an area, the sense of community, and social capital. Shaw explains in detail each of these distinct ways that neighborhoods can affect health and notes that "the housing people live in, and the environment in which that housing is located, is considered in physical, social and, cultural terms." She also notes that because housing, health and poverty are so interconnected with one another, it is difficult to disentangle effects and prove specific and direct casual links among them. Shaw's matrix is important in organizing the different pathways by which housing quality, and ultimately, neighborhood quality, can affect health outcomes.

Material housing conditions within neighborhoods can directly affect maternal health. For example, general housing damage, such as poor insulation or broken windows, can affect respiratory health as a result of inadequate control of temperature, moisture, and ventilation (3). Yet, while current research does seem to demonstrate a significant relationship between the direct physical effects of housing quality and health outcomes, the focus of this review is to examine the literature on the influences of the wider spatial environment within the neighborhood context and its relationship to birth weight. A high level of physical disorder in a neighborhood may signal that social control in the neighborhood is deteriorating (8). A study by Ross-Mirowsky (2001) surveyed a random sample of Illinois residents and found that residents who reported higher levels of physical disorder in their neighborhood, such as graffiti or abandoned buildings, also reported significantly worse health even after adjusting for individual socioeconomic disadvantage (15). It appears then that a mechanism by which neighborhood environments can influence maternal health is through maternal stress.

Maternal stress and birth weight

A clear connection exists between psychosocial stress and poor birth outcomes, which include both preterm delivery and low birth weight (16,17). Klebanoff defined a stressor as "any physical or psychological demand or challenge that alters or has the potential to alter the internal milieu of the organism in homeostasis" (18). He goes on to explain that stressors among people may vary from major life events such as divorce or death of a relative, to daily concerns and worries that may include financial, employment or family related matters. In this paper we focus on the chronic stressors related to a poor neighborhood environment.

Physiological responses to stressors in the environment is mediated by the hypothalamus-pituitary adrenal cortex system (HPA axis) (19). When a person is exposed to a stressor, large quantities of stress hormones, including corticotropin-releasing hormone (CRH) and adrenaline are released into the circulatory system. The hormones then act as signals that induce bodily responses in mothers that can result in reduction in blood flow to the uterus and fetus along with stress-induced release of placental CRH to the intrauterine environment. Reduced blood flow to the uterus and fetus can result in intrauterine growth retardation where the fetal weight is significantly below the normal weight for gestational age. Stress in expectant mothers may also result in high fetal cortisol that can lead to poor placental function, further inhibiting growth and development (20). Furthermore, a study by Rich-Edwards and Grizzard (2005) found a correlation between high placental cortisol levels and spontaneous preterm delivery (21).

The effects of chronic neighborhood stress may also increase the risk of preterm birth via psychological distress, and especially via the development of a depressive self-concept (17, 22). Kramer defines the depressive self-concept as "depression about one's current state, dissatisfaction with life, as well as a sense of hopelessness and a lack of optimism about the future" (23). Depression during pregnancy has been linked to adverse pregnancy outcomes, including low birth weight and growth retardation (22). Kramer goes on to say that depression may induce mothers to perceive common challenges with a heightened sense of stress, creating a cycle whereby stress reinforces the depression. The depression may thus trigger a physiological response that can contribute to the release of stress hormones. Mothers may also engage in coping behaviors, such as the use of cigarettes or alcohol, which increase the risk of preterm birth and low birth weight (10).

Continuous chronic exposure to stressors like anxiety over poor living conditions or high crime levels exacerbates the effects of acute stress as can be found when examining allostatic load. While homeostasis refers to the internal processes of the body that regulate its response to challenges and demands, allostasis refers to the process of the body's response to those challenges (24). An example of an allostatic process is the fight or flight response that the body may experience when it encounters a stressor in the form of a challenge of perceived danger (25). Frequent activation of the body's stress response, such as if the body is chronically exposed to excessive demands in its environment, may cause adverse long term consequences on physiological mechanisms, in that the regulatory system may lose its ability to effectively respond to those demands and protect the body against harm (24). This further supports the idea that neighborhood environments and living conditions in which individuals spend the majority of their time have a significant impact on health.

Besides the effects of stress hormones on physiological responses in the body, maternal stress may also lead to destructive coping behaviors such as alcohol use and smoking that is directly related to low birth weight (26). While significant consumption of alcohol during pregnancy may result in Fetal Alcohol Syndrome (FAS), which is characterized by growth retardation and cognitive defects, moderate alcohol drinking may have similar consequences in Fetal Alcohol Effects (FAE) which is associated with intrauterine growth retardation and spontaneous preterm delivery (27). One of the most influential maternal behavioral mechanisms that result in low birth weight is cigarette smoking (28). Cigarette smoke contains an assortment of potentially harmful chemicals that can include carbon monoxide, cyanide compounds and other toxins that can inhibit fetal growth (28). Cigarettes also contain nicotine that can not only act as an appetite suppressant that can hinder a healthy diet for the mother, resulting in low nutrients and low birth weight in the infant, but it can also increase the release of maternal stress hormones that can consequently constrict blood flow to the fetus (26).

Social capital as a mediating factor of stress

The ability of people to adapt to stressful environments may depend on their access to informal resources such as social relationships and institutions that generate social capital (29). Social capital is typically thought of as the social ties among persons and positions. Putnam (30) defined social capital as "features of social organization, such as networks, norms, and trust, that facilitate coordination and cooperation for mutual benefit." Neighborhoods in which residents are engaged in their community's social life are more likely to offer social support that can help mediate the effects of external environmental stressors (31). Residents may aid one another with everyday tasks, such as childcare or monitoring each other's property. In contrast, a relative lack of neighborhood support has been found to be a risk factor for low birth weight even after adjusting for individual maternal risk factors (31,32).

Measures of crime, vacancy, and tenure can serve as helpful indicators of neighborhood social capital (33). Areas with high concentrations of vacant houses and renter-occupied tenants (as opposed to owner-occupied) have little residential stability and may not provide an important buffer to the deleterious effects of increased stress levels on health. Furthermore, high levels of crime may raise distrust among residents, reducing social capital and increasing stress (34, 35). Perceptions of disorder and lack of social capital have been associated with maternal stress, which may in turn lead to alcohol and tobacco use, both of which can adversely affect birth weight (36).

According to Shaw (3) "[P]eople do not just live in houses: They live in and experience neighborhoods." For expectant mothers, unfavorable perceptions of their residential environment may be associated with low birth weight for their infants (37). Appropriate measures of neighborhood quality are therefore needed in order to understand how mothers may perceive their surroundings to elucidate the role that residential environments may play in relation to low birth weight.

Traditional and proposed measures of neighborhood quality

The majority of the current literature utilizes data from the US Census on Population and Housing and resident questionnaires to measure neighborhood quality. Such measures may include census statistics describing rates of poverty, unemployment and residential stability to develop an index for neighborhood quality (38-40). For example, a study by Matheson (39) used census tract characteristics that identified two measures of neighborhood chronic stress: residential mobility and material deprivation. Residential instability was measured by examining characteristics such as percentage home ownership, percentage moving within the last 5 years, and percentage married. Material deprivation was measured looking at high school graduation, percentage of lone parent families, percentage of families receiving government transfer payments and percentage living below the poverty rate. Yet socioeconomic demographics are only one dimension of neighborhood characteristics and tend to describe characteristics of the neighborhood's residents rather than of the physical features of the neighborhood itself.

Therefore, there is a need for the development of an objective and record-based approach that takes into account observable physical variables to determine neighborhood quality (41). To create the groundwork for these necessary methods, Sampson and Raudenbush conducted a study to examine physical disorder in neighborhoods (42). In 1999, they employed researchers to collect observational assessments by driving a vehicle at a rate of five miles per hour down every street in 196 Chicago census tracts (42).

The unit of analysis was a block face, defined as each block segment on one side of the street. Each vehicle had a pair of video recorders on each side of the vehicle in order to capture social activities and physical features present within the block faces on opposite sides of the street. While the cameras were recording, two trained observers, one on each side of the vehicle, made note of presences of harmful items along the street. They coded the analysis with 1 = presence and 0 = absence of the indicator of disorder. The ten scale items included such things as the presence or absence of cigarettes in the street, garbage or litter, and empty beer bottles. Sampson and Raudenbush took the first step to create a scale to measure physical disorder that furthered the understanding of how to objectively collect information about neighborhood quality. Their method of collecting data through video recordings was a rough observation strategy that was limited to ten variables, which are not enough to provide a comprehensive profile of the neighborhood's physical built environment.

A more accurate and robust measure of the neighborhood built environment might thus be developed in order to better assess neighborhood quality and its relationship to birth weight. As defined earlier, the built environment is comprised of the physical conditions of the home, in addition to other buildings, spaces and products that are created or modified by people (6). Future built environment measures should therefore not only take into account the structural integrity of the neighborhood's residential homes, but also the spatial proximity of neighborhood amenities. Furthermore, similar to Sampson and Raudenbush's recording of physical disorder in the neighborhoods, measures of litter and physical eyesores associated with stressful neighborhood conditions should also be recorded to provide a more complete assessment of the built environment.

A review of the literature demonstrates that maternal stress has been linked to negative birth outcomes, including low birth weight (16-18). As depicted in the cycle of disadvantage and disability, the built environment has the potential to act through the pathways of maternal stress and low self-worth to induce negative birth outcomes that can carry on into future childhood development (20, 21). Yet while there has been some research examining the link between a poor built environment and stress in residents, evaluations of neighborhood conditions are based on residents' perceptions. As a result, the direction of causation between residents' self-reported stress and the self-reported conditions of the neighborhood may be skewed.

INTERVENTIONS

Low birth weight is only one of many negative health outcomes, including obesity and diabetes, which may be negatively affected by the built environment (43). Developing more accurate measures of the built environment may not only be helpful in examining relationships of neighborhoods to birth weight, but other the effects of neighborhood environments on other health outcomes. More accurate, objective measures of the built environment may assist community leaders and policy in designing maps that could help track vulnerable areas, thus aiding in the development of intervention strategies to specifically target those areas most in need.

Interventions aimed at breaking the cycle of the built environment and low birth weight can be implemented at the county, neighborhood and individual levels. At the county level, policymakers can make zoning changes that could promote higher quality affordable housing. Raising housing quality standards might translate into better health for residents in homes as well as the neighborhood.

Interventions at the neighborhood level can also be implemented to mediate the adverse effects of the built environment. Neighborhood level change can include collaborative partnerships among people and organizations from different sectors, such as schools and businesses, working together to improve the health and welfare of residents (44). Collaborative partnerships within the neighborhoods can draw from a multitude of resources to address the unique challenges of the specific communities they serve. For example, locals banks and community organizations might work together to promote homeownership and economic opportunity for vulnerable populations. Local non-profit agencies might offer low-interests loans and help borrowers to build wealth through ownership of a home or business by enabling private lenders to make loans in low-wealth communities. Thus, underserved communities can be strengthened through the financing of nonprofits, childcare centers and community health facilities, which can serve as neighborhood resources for those in need (44, 45)

At the clinical level, neighborhoods may be identified where there is a high risk for environmental stressors. Health providers can then allocate specific resources for those mothers that may need more support. They may also provide increased care coordination, which has been demonstrated to increase pregnant mothers' resilience to stressors, leading to better birth outcomes (46-48). Because, many mothers have difficulty navigating the health care system to find nutritional, medical, education and financial resources, care coordination would include transportation and assistance along with follow-up and mentoring and counseling to helping mothers secure the support they need.

CONCLUSION

Perceived physical disorder in the neighborhood's built environment has been demonstrated to elevate fear and anxiety in residents. Signs of neighborhood disorder, like vandalism and graffiti, can serve as cues that social control in the neighborhood is deteriorating. Concerns about crime and safety may thus expose pregnant mothers to high levels of stress, resulting in poor health and harmful coping mechanisms that can lead to negative birth outcomes, including low birth weight.

Because the effects of environmentally driven disparities are likely manifested in a multi-phase cycle, there are numerous stages at which interventions can be implemented at the county, neighborhood and individual level to break the cycle of disadvantage and disability brought on by a poor neighborhood built environment.

ACKNOWLEDGMENTS

I would like to acknowledge Martha Keating, MS, Pamela J Maxson, PhD, Marie Lynn Miranda, PhD, and Gretchen Kroeger, MEM for their mentorship during this project. This chapter is an updated and revised version of the original publication: Quyang R The relationship between the built environment and birth weight. Rev Environ Health 2011;26(3):181-6.

REFERENCES

[1]   Hodgson M. Indoor environmental, exposures and symptoms. Environ Health Perspect Suppl 2002:663.

[2]   Saegert SC, Klitzman S, Freudenberg N, Cooperman-Mroczek J, Nassar S. Healthy housing: A structured review of published evaluations of US interventions to improve health by modifying housing in the United States, 1990-2001. Am J Public Health 2003;93(9):1471-7.

[3]   Shaw M. Housing and public health. Annu Rev Public Health 2004;25(1):397-418.

[4]   Jackson RJ. The impact of the built environment on health: An emerging field. Am J Public Health 2003;93(9):1382-4.

[5]   Wilhelm M. Outdoor air pollution, family and neighborhood environment, and asthma in LA FANS children.(Report) Report. Health Place 2009;15(1):25.

[6]   Srinivasan S, O'Fallon LR, Dearry A. Creating healthy communities, healthy homes, healthy people: Initiating a research agenda on the built environment and public health. Am J Public Health 2003;93(9):1446-50.

[7]   Ross CE, Mirowsky J. Disorder and decay - The concept and measurement of perceived neighborhood disorder. Urban Affairs Rev 1999;34(3):412-32.

[8]   Hill TD, Ross CE, Angel RJ. Neighborhood disorder, psychophysiological distress, and health. J Health Soc Behav 2005;46(2):170-86.

[9]   Latkin CA, Curry AD. Stressful neighborhoods and depression: A prospective study of the impact of neighborhood disorder. J Health Soc Behav 2003;44(1):34-44.

[10]   Nordentoft M, Lou HC, Hansen D, Nim J, Pyrds O, Rubin P, et al. Intrauterine growth retardation and premature delivery: The influence of maternal smoking and psychosocial factors. Am J Public Health 1996;86(3):347-54.

[11]   Horbar JD, Badger GJ, Carpenter JH, Fanaroff AA, Kilpatrick S, LaCorte M, et al. Trends in mortality and morbidity for very low birth weight infants, 1991-1999. Pediatrics 2002;110(1):143-51.

[12]   Hack M, Klein NK, Taylor HG. Long-term developmental outcomes of low birth weight infants. Future Children 1995;5(1):176-96.

[13]   Datar A, Jacknowitz A. Birth weight effects on children's mental, motor, and physical development: Evidence from twins data. Maternal Child Health J 2009;13(6):780-94.

[14]   Paneth NS. The problem of low birth weight. Future Children 1995;5(1):19-34.

[15]   Ross C, John M. Neighborhood disadvantage, disorder, and health. J Health Soc Behav 2001;42(3):258-76.

[16]   Wadhwa PD, Sandman CA, Porto M, Dunkelschetter C, Garite TJ. The association between prenatal stress and infant birth weight and gestational age at birth: A prospective investigation. Am J Obstet Gynecol 1993;169(4):858-65.

[17]   Copper RL, Goldenberg RL, Das A, Elder N, Swain M, Norman G, et al. The preterm prediction study: Maternal stress is associated with spontaneous preterm birth at less than thirty-five weeks' gestation. Am J Obstet Gynecol 1996;175(5):1286-92.

[18]   Klebanoff MA. Psychosocial stress in pregnany and infancy worskhop. Bethesda, MD, 2003. Accessed 2013 May 10. URL: http://www.nationalchildrensstudy.gov/ research/workshops/Pages/preg_report112003.aspx.

[19]   Mulder EJH, Robles de Medina PG, Huizink AC, Van den Bergh BRH, Buitelaar JK, Visser GHA. Prenatal maternal stress: effects on pregnancy and the (unborn) child. Early Hum Dev 2002;70(1-2):3-14.

[20]   Gitau RC, A. Fisk, N.M., Glover, V. Fetal exposure to maternal cortisol. Lancet 1998;352(9129):707-8.

[21]   Rich-Edwards JW, Grizzard TA. Psychosocial stress and neuroendocrine mechanisms in preterm delivery. Am J Obstet Gynecol 2005;192(5):S30-S5.

[22]   Chung TKH, Lau TK, Yip ASK, Chiu HFK, Lee DTS. Antepartum depressive symptomatology is associated with adverse obstetric and neonatal outcomes. Psychosom Med 2001;63(5):830-4.

[23]   Kramer MS, Seguin L, Lydon J, Goulet L. Socio-economic disparities in pregnancy outcome: why do the poor fare so poorly. Paediatr Perinatal Epidemiol 2000;14:194-210.

[24]   McEwen B. Stress and the individual: mechanisms leading to disease. Arch Intern Med 1993;153(2093):101.

[25]   McEwen BS. Physiology and neurobiology of stress and adaptation: Central role of the brain. Physiol Rev 2007;87(3):873-904.

[26]   Kramer MS. Determinants of low birth weight: methodological assessment and meta-analysis. Bull World Health Organ 1987 1987;65(5):663-737.

[27]   Ornoy A, Ergaz Z. Alcohol abuse in pregnant women: Effects on the fetus and newborn, mode of action and maternal treatment. Int J Environ Res Public Health 2010;7(2):364-79.

[28]   Shea AK, Steiner M. Cigarette smoking during pregnancy. Nicotine Tobacco Res 2008;10(2):267-78.

[29]   Anderson NB, Bulatao RA, Cohen B, National Research Council. Panel on race and health in later life. Critical perspectives on racial and ethnic differences in health in late life: Washington, DC: National Academies Press, 2004.

[30]   Putnam R. The prosperous community: Social capital and community life. Am Prospect 1993;4(13):35-42.

[31]   Boardman JD. Stress and physical health: the role of neighborhoods as mediating and moderating mechanisms. Soc Sci Med 2004;58(12):2473.

[32]   Buka SL, Brennan RT, Rich-Edwards JW, Raudenbush SW, Earls F. Neighborhood support and the birth weight of urban infants. Am J Epidemiol 2003;157(1):1-8.

[33]   Sampson RJ, Graif C. Neighborhood social capital as differential social organization: Resident and leadership dimensions. Am Behav Scientist 2009;52(11):1579-605.

[34]   Masi CM, Hawkley LC, Harry Piotrowski Z, Pickett KE. Neighborhood economic disadvantage, violent crime, group density, and pregnancy outcomes in a diverse, urban population. Soc Sci Med 2007;65(12):2440-57.

[35]   Sampson RJ, Raudenbush SW. Neighborhoods and violent crime: A multilevel study of collective efficacy. Science 1997;277(5328):918.

[36]   Moiduddin E, Massey DS. Neighborhood disadvantage and birth weight: The role of perceived danger and substance abuse. Int J Conflict Violence 2008;2(1):113-29.

[37]   James W. Collins, Jr., Richard JD, Rebecca S, Arden H, Stephen W, Steven A. African-American mothers' perception of their residential environment, stressful life events, and very low birthweight. Epidemiol 1998;9(3):286-9.

[38]   O'Campo P, Xiaonan X, Mei-Cheng W, Caughy MOB. Neighborhood risk factors for low birthweight in Baltimore: A multilevel analysis. Am J Public Health 1997;87(7):1113-8.

[39]   Matheson FI, Moineddin R, Dunn JR, Creatore MI, Gozdyra P, Glazier RH. Urban neighborhoods, chronic stress, gender and depression. Soc Sci Med 2006;63(10):2604-16.

[40]   Roberts EM. Neighborhood social environments and the distribution of low birthweight in Chicago. Am J Public Health 1997;87(4):597-603.

[41]   Thomson H, Petticrew M, Morrison D. Health effects of housing improvement: systematic review of intervention studies. BMJ 2001;323(7306):187-90.

[42]   Sampson RJ, Raudenbush SW. Systematic social observation of public spaces: A new look at disorder in urban neighborhoods. Am J Sociol 1999;105(3):603.

[43]   Singh GK, Siahpush M, Kogan MD. Neighborhood socioeconomic conditions, built environments, and childhood obesity. Health Affairs 2010;29(3):503-12.

[44]   Roussos ST, Fawcett SB. A review of collaborative partnerships as a strategy for improving community health. Annu Rev Public Health 2000;21(1):369-402.

[45]   Altschuler A, Somkin CP, Adler NE. Local services and amenities, neighborhood social capital, and health. Soc Sci Med 2004;59(6):1219-29.

[46]   Canning PM, Frizzell LM, Courage ML. Birth outcomes associated with prenatal participation in a government support programme for mothers with low incomes. Child Care Health Dev 2009;36(2):225-31.

[47]   Ricketts SA, Murray EK, Schwalberg R. Reducing low birthweight by resolving risks: Results from Colorado's Prenatal Plus Program. Am J Public Health 2005;95(11):1952-7.

[48]   Baldwin L-M, Larson EH, Connell FA, Nordlund D, Cain KC, Cawthon ML, et al. The effect of expanding Medicaid prenatal services on birth outcomes. Am J Public Health 1998;88(11):1623-9.

In: Born into this World: Health Issues
Editors: D. E. Greydanus, A. N. Feinberg et al.

ISBN: 978-1-63321-667-9
© 2014 Nova Science Publishers, Inc.

Chapter 9

CYCLE OF ENVIRONMENTAL HEALTH DISPARITIES

*I Leslie Rubin, MD**

Department of Pediatrics, Morehouse School of Medicine and Innovative
Solutions for Disadvantage and Disability, Atlanta, Georgia,
United States of America

The health of individuals and populations of individuals is not uniform, consistent or equitable. There are differences in the health of populations between different countries and there are differences in the health of groups of people within any specific country. These differences do not necessarily relate to the inherent predisposition of any one person or group of people to adverse health conditions, but rather to factors that are often beyond their control. These factors are significantly influenced by: political and economic forces of a country that determine the availability and distribution of healthcare and other related resources; social and cultural practices and mores that further shape differences in the health status; and, other personal and environmental factors in homes, neighborhoods and communities; together these factors constitute the social determinants of health (SDH). This complex array of influences combines to translate into health disparities experienced by people within and between countries across the globe. In this chapter we will examine

---

* Correspondence: I Leslie Rubin, MD, Research Associate Professor, Department of Pediatrics, Morehouse School of Medicine and President, Innovative Solutions for Disadvantage and Disability, 776 Windsor Parkway, Atlanta, GA 30342, United States. E-mail: lrubi01@emory.edu

the concepts of social determinants of health and of health disparities as they relate to children and adults with intellectual and developmental disabilities (IDD).

INTRODUCTION

In the traditional medical mindset, we have the notion that a person is generally well, becomes ill, seeks medical attention, is treated and returns to good health. This model, long part of the traditional western healthcare delivery system, does not adequately address the realities that determine underlying health status, factors that determine health and well-being of individuals or groups of individuals, and does not recognize the realities of chronic conditions that require a more complex approach. In order to begin to examine these concepts it is important to explore the factors that determine the health and well-being of population groups, and how this impacts the health and functioning of individuals and of families.

The term Social Determinants of Health (SDH) refers to the conditions in which people are born, grow, play, learn, work, live, and age. The expression of these factors can be seen reflected in statistics on the health of populations, for example the infant mortality rate (IMR), which is often used as an indicator of the level of health in a country. It is measured by the number of deaths of infants less than one year of age per 1,000 live births. The worldwide infant mortality rate is 49.4, according to the United Nations.

Countries that enjoy good overall health and good healthcare tend to have low IMR, such as Sweden with an IMR of 2.6, Singapore at 2.53, the UK at 4.44 and the United States at a rate of 6.17. By contrast, with healthcare systems that are less developed, the IMR is high, for example Turkey where the IMR is 21.43 and South Africa where it is 41.61. The highest scores are those of Somalia at 100.14, and Afghanistan, where the IMR is a staggering 117.23 (1). Perhaps it is not coincidental that these countries have long been engaged in armed conflict.

In countries where there is political tension, or worse, armed conflict, there is suffering. Not only to the combatants, but innocent civilians are also affected, resulting in physical and emotional injuries, while infrastructure that assures the availably and distribution of food, healthcare and other resources to citizens is disrupted if not devastated. Wars result in dramatic increases in mortality of populations along with the physical and emotional disabilities that result (2).

During the conflict in the Balkans in the mid 1990's, the Gypsies of Kosovo, who had thrived in the region for almost 150 years, were attacked and displaced. Families were placed in refugee camps that were located near a lead mine and smelting works. The factory had been closed, but left behind a veritable mountain of toxic lead waste. The exposure of the children to high amounts of lead causing severe toxicity, which resulted in high morbidity and mortality of the children (3). Unfortunately, the damage has been done and continues to be a problem, in significant part because the people represent a minority community who are disenfranchised.

SOCIAL DETERMINANTS OF HEALTH

The World Health Organization (WHO) defines social determinants of health as the complex, integrated, and overlapping social structures and economic systems that are responsible for most health inequities. These social structures and economic systems include the social environment, physical environment, health services, and structural and societal factors (4). Social determinants of health are shaped by the distribution of money, power, and resources throughout local communities, nations, and the world.

The WHO has focused on the social determinants of health as a means to achieve the millennium development goals (MDG) of the United Nations (UN). The MDG are a set of eight goals, established in 2000 and set to be achieved by 2015, to eradicate extreme poverty and hunger; achieve universal primary education; reduce child mortality; promote gender equality and improve maternal health; combat HIV/AIDS, malaria, and other diseases; ensure environmental sustainability; and, develop a global partnership for development (5). This blueprint, agreed to by all the world's countries and all the world's leading development institutions, outlines a set of themes that are integral to global plan as it moves forward. Each of these factors may be viewed independently or as being interrelated, and together they represent the set of factors that require attention of everyone concerned about the health of individuals, communities and populations:

- Employment conditions – this refers to the ability of citizens to work and earn money to support themselves and their families. It follows that unemployment means lack of resources to feed, clothe and house families and can result in malnutrition and increased susceptibility to illness

- Social exclusion – refers to the discrimination of one group of people by another resulting in the inability of the excluded group to access resources available to others in the same community or society
- Priority public health conditions – this refers to the role of public health in developing programs that that increase access to healthcare for socially and economically disadvantaged groups.
- Women and gender equity – in many societies, women have a lower status than men in accessing resources. This is a critical element in the determination of the health of children from conception, through vulnerabilities during pregnancy and to the care and support during childhood. Remediation of this aspect needs a focus on the appreciation of the concept of maternal and child health
- Early child development – this element is critical in establishing physical, emotional and social well-being for children to assure that they will grow up to be healthy and become fully participating and contributing citizens.
- Globalization – this phenomenon illustrates the interconnection between countries and how relationships between countries can affect the health of its citizens through the economics of trade and through the sharing of resources.
- Health systems – this is a critical element in assuring the health of individuals and populations through public health programs and through the availability and accessibly of healthcare resources
- Measurement and evidence – this element represents the importance of research and constant examination of existing and changing circumstances towards improvement of services to improve the health of communities and societies.
- Urbanization – in the global context, this refers to the movement of people from rural areas to cities, in search of opportunities and in search of sustenance. This phenomenon results in poor living conditions that in turn result in poor health conditions.

The phenomenon of urbanization dates back to the period of the industrial revolution and was captured by Charles Dickens (1812-1870), who wrote about the burden of being poor in 19th century London. In that early age of industrialization, as exists in our current times, advances in technology brought dramatic progress to society; at the same time it caused seismic shifts in populations from rural agricultural settings and lifestyles, to the cities, where the new engines of industry promised more opportunities. Unfortunately, it also resulted in overcrowding, disenfranchisement and poverty for many, highlighting the contrasts between those who benefitted from the advances in industrialization and those who suffered as a consequence. Katherine Boo, in her book, "Behind the beautiful everlastings", captured the plight of people living in the slums of Mumbai in the end of the first decade of the 21st century (6). She describes the lives of people who populated Annawadi, a makeshift settlement in the shadow of luxury hotels near the Mumbai airport. In a 2001 census, it was estimated that about 6.5 million people were living in the slums of Mumbai representing nearly 55% of Mumbai's population. It has been estimated that in 2011 there were 8 million people living in the slums (7). The numbers are staggering, and the sense of despair and fragile hope is captured by Boo in her chronicle.

The similarities between late 19th century London and early 21st century Mumbai are striking. Although the differences are those of time, place and order of magnitude, both contrast the affluence of the world outside with the world of poverty, environmental hazards, and emotional stress, distress and suffering.

In a poor rural area of Nigeria, illegal gold mining using children to perform much of the labor resulted in 'an outbreak of childhood lead poisoning with child mortality unprecedented in modern times'. Investigators found that the children came in direct contact with large amounts of lead through daily activities, which provided a constant and direct route of exposure to lead for these children. The level of exposure was so high that 25% of the children under the age of 5 years died as a result of exposure and 97% of the surviving children required chelation therapy (8)

Unfortunately, this type of artisanal and small-scale mining (ASM) is occurring on a global scale. According to the Global Mercury Project, an initiative of the United Nations, ASM occurs in more than 55 countries, and 10–15 million miners work in ASM operations globally, primarily in Africa, Asia, and South America. An estimated 100 million people globally rely directly or indirectly on ASM for their livelihood (9). For many individuals, participation in mining is driven by poverty and a lack of economic opportunities, especially in rural communities, as seen in this outbreak.

Lead toxicity is the most common environmental cause of brain damage and its consequences on development and function. Children who are poor and to live in older houses where there is more likely to be residual lead-based paint, are almost four times more likely to have lead toxicity with its consequent effect on learning, cognition and behavior. The WHO estimates that lead poisoning causes 0.6% of the global burden of disease and contributes to approximately 600,000 cases of intellectual disability in children annually (10). Although lead has largely been outlawed from paint and gasoline in the US and other countries, it still exits and in fact dramatic episodes have been reported around overwhelming lead toxicity in children that resulted in significant mortality as well as morbidly for the poor, unemployed and marginalized populations, as was the case of the children in Nigeria described above.

HEALTH DISPARITIES

Health disparity is defined by the CDC (Centers for Disease Control and Prevention) as a difference in health that is closely linked with social or economic disadvantage. Health disparities negatively affect groups of people who have systematically experienced greater social or economic obstacles to health. These obstacles stem from characteristics historically linked to discrimination or exclusion such as race or ethnicity, religion, socioeconomic status, gender, mental health, sexual orientation, or geographic location. Other characteristics include cognitive, sensory, or physical disability (11).

Health disparities are preventable differences in the burden of disease, injury, violence, or opportunities to achieve optimal health that are experienced by socially disadvantaged populations and result from multiple factors:

- Poverty
- Environmental threats
- Inadequate access to health care
- Educational inequalities
- Individual and behavioral factors

There are significant health disparities among people who live in poverty, in part because poor people tend to live in areas where there may be more toxins from factories and other industrial plants that are more likely to be located in or near poorer neighborhoods whose population is often marginalized and relatively disenfranchised with less financial and political capital. This is exemplified in the situation of Anniston Alabama in the late part of the 20th century (12).

The town of Anniston Alabama had its start in the late 19th Century as a mining town and rapidly grew. Soon, however, foundries sprang up and gave way to industry and chemical manufacturing, including a military chemical weapons development site in the area.

For the first half of the 20th Century and in the immediate post-World War II decades, the town of Anniston flourished economically. There were jobs and there were opportunities. However, as early as the 1970s, pollution was noted in the rivers and streams, and over the next two decades as more and heavier pollution was identified, the Agency for Toxic Substances and Disease Registry (ATSDR) of the CDC was called on to conduct a survey of Polychlorinated Biphenyl (PCB) levels in the affected areas (11). The levels of PCB in the population were found to be in the high toxic range. The affected citizenry was outraged and lawsuits against the chemical companies began to appear. As the citizens' action groups became more vocal, increasing national attention was being focused on the pollution and on the legal battles. In the meantime, the chemical companies, sensing the situation, closed their operations in Anniston, and, with the closure and departure of the factories and associated industries and businesses, the economy of the town suffered. There were not as many jobs and with the loss of the tax base, and public services suffered as well. This left the affected citizens without jobs, without a dependable source of income and vulnerable to the effect of poverty, unemployment and the consequent social and health implications.

VULNERABILITY OF CHILDREN

Children are more vulnerable to environmental factors than adults because they are in the process of physiological growth and change, they have a higher metabolic rate, they drink more water and eat more food in relation to their body weight, and their organs are growing and developing, especially their brains (13).

Furthermore, children from poor areas live in neighborhoods that are not safe, have limited resources, limited access to recreational areas and green space, and have limited access to healthy foods, limited opportunities for guided recreation by family or other adults, and are more likely to sit at home and watch television. These factors predispose children to obesity (14) and the significant related health consequences, such as hypertension, diabetes and sleep apnea, conditions that affect academic performance in school, with a greater likelihood of having emotional difficulties and mental health problems such as depression.

Children who are poor are also more likely to have asthma (15). It is more likely that their parents or other family members will smoke and will live in houses with more dust, more mold and malfunctioning heating and air-conditioning systems, which affects the indoor air quality. The mortality of asthma in poor children is much greater than for their more affluent counterparts (16).

Related to these disproportionate presentations of acute and chronic conditions, families who are poor are more likely to rely on public health insurance (Medicaid in the US), have limited access to quality healthcare with inconsistent attention by a primary care pediatrician, and are more likely to be admitted to the hospital for inpatient treatment or to use the emergency room (ER) for healthcare (15,17). The use of the ER for health care is not only inadequate for optional health but unnecessarily increases the cost of health care.

For this group of children and adolescences, their schools are more likely to be in disrepair, and they are more likely to have a poorer education, more likely to have school difficulties, to be absent from school, to have learning and behavior difficulties and to be suspended or drop out of school and to be unemployed at age 24 years (18). They also are more likely to join gangs, engage in risky and violent behaviors (19), and have difficulties with substance abuse. These behaviors for males result in an increased likelihood for arrest and incarceration and for the females, sexual activity and the risk of pregnancy (20). For both men and women, there is grave concern for sexually transmitted diseases especially for HIV/AIDS. In fact, concern about prevalence and transmission HIV/AIDS is greatest in this population (21).

For young women living in poverty who become pregnant, they may continue with their substance abuse during pregnancy, and are less likely to seek prenatal care and take care of themselves. As a result, they are more likely to have premature infants. These premature infants are then more likely to be smaller and have more neonatal problems (22). When these babies eventually leave the hospital and go home, they are less likely to receive optimal positive stimulation and early intervention services. Accordingly, they are more likely to have intellectual and developmental disabilities (IDD), which will tend to be more severe and they will be less likely to have appropriate intervention services and therefore a poorer outcome. Furthermore, these young women may not be able to take care of their children, particularly if the infants are irritable and have additional healthcare and developmental needs. These mothers are more likely to have difficulty managing their children and, because they are young and have significant difficulties of their own, there is a greater likelihood of neglect and abuse, such as shaken baby syndrome or head injury which can result in serious consequences with brain damage. In addition, these infants and children are more likely to be referred to social services and be placed in foster care or in the care of another family member, often the grandparent (23).

TOXIC STRESS FOR CHILDREN

For children growing up under these circumstances, the daily stresses of life can take their toll. Schonkoff and colleagues have conceptualized the phenomenon of stress in children and translated it into a classification that has real physiological, emotional and social implications not only for the health of the children, but with significant health implications when they grow into adulthood (24). They categorized stress into three levels, the first being the inevitable day to day stresses of life as encountered by poor and rich children alike. Having to separate from parents and go to school, having to learn, to deal with social ups and downs, to have illnesses, to go to the doctor and have injections, and, in general, to be disappointed every now and then, and at times to have emotional distress about relationships. These day to day stresses are part of growing up and learning about life, and as long as there is a supportive parent around to help deal with the situations, the child will overcome the temporary adversity and go forward, learn from the experience and perhaps be better for it.

The second level of stress occurs when there is a major life experience of a singular and dramatic nature, such as a death in the family, a move of residence, a natural disaster, a parental divorce, or a major social setback. Again, the finite nature of the event, the return to a reasonable level of predictability in life, and the resumption of pattern of behavior with strong parental support will enable the child to most likely overcome the emotional impact of the experience, learn from it and perhaps become more resilient.

The third level of stress has a pattern of chronicity and relentlessness, in repeated and multiple insults and stresses with limited, inadequate or unpredictable nurturing, support and guidance of a parent or caring adult. In fact, at times, in the case of child abuse in its various forms, the reliance and trust that children naturally have with the relevant adults in their lives, is broken beyond repair. The consequences of these levels of stress and insult are then codified into the child's brain and physiology as well as psyche, and not only adversely affect the child's health and ability to deal with life, but also have implications on that child's physical emotional and social wellbeing into adulthood. These adverse childhood experiences are associated with adverse health outcomes as adults that also result in reduced life expectancy. This level is termed toxic stress (24).

DISPARITIES AND INTELLECTUAL DISABILITY

Children who grow up in poverty with the stresses of food insecurity, insecurity about where they will live, fear of abuse, fear of crime on the streets, environments with litter, noise and broken windows, families in constant transition, flux and motion, changing schools and other adverse environmental factors in the home, in the neighborhood, at schools and at play are more likely to have learning disabilities, attention deficit/hyperactivity disorder (ADHD), and IDD, which may be undiagnosed, misdiagnosed, and/or untreated (25,26). Also, they are less likely to actually be diagnosed with an autism spectrum disorder (ASD) (27) and misdiagnosed with a variety of other conditions, including conduct disorder or oppositional defiant disorder. Both these latter diagnoses carry significant prejudicial attitudes and make it less likely that these children will receive appropriate services for their ASD and more likely to be treated with neuroleptic medication, while their real needs are neglected or overlooked. Children in foster care are more likely to be treated with psychotropic medications, which can have serious side effects (28). Cerebral palsy (CP) is more common among low income and minority populations (29). This is mainly attributable to the higher incidence of prematurity among the poor, less educated and minority population who may be in their teenage years.

A survey of children attending a CP clinic in downtown Atlanta in the early part of the millennium revealed a population of children who were predominantly African American, poor, receiving services through the state funded Title V programs for "Children with special health care needs" (CSHCN). The survey revealed significant medical complexity, but most striking were the demographics and psychosocial findings. Many of the children were born prematurely with a maternal history of substance abuse (tobacco, alcohol or other drugs) with a direct correlation of degree of prematurity with maternal substance abuse (see figure 1). Furthermore, approximately 50% of the children were living with single mothers, another 20

% with their grandmothers and about 10% in foster homes. The remaining 20% were living in two parent families and tended to have been born at term (see figure 2).

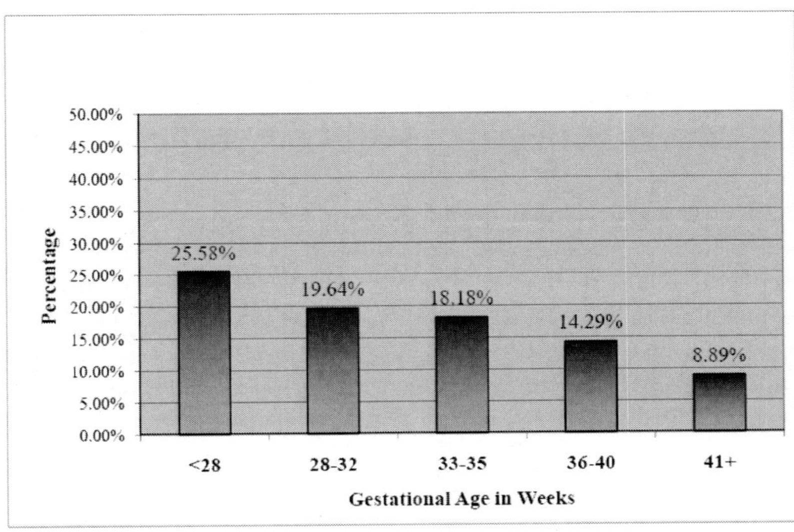

Figure 1. Percentage of patients whose mothers used substances during pregnancy, per gestational age group.

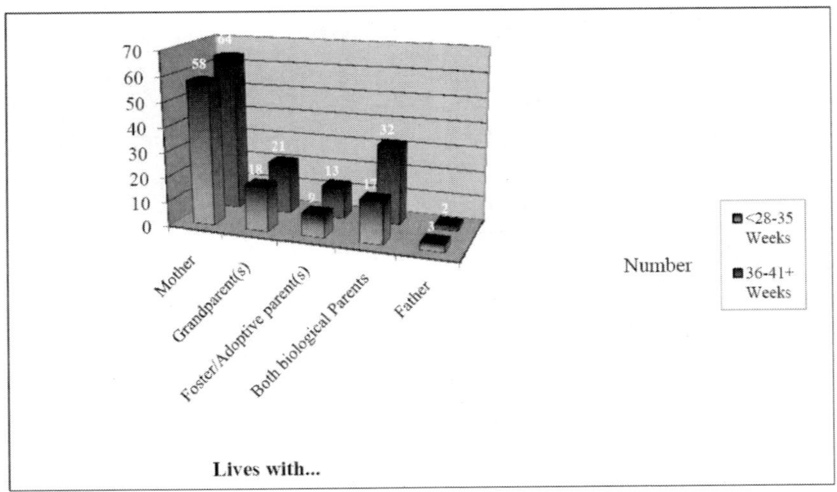

Figure 2. With whom the patient lives by gestational age, in weeks.

This pattern of a social substrate of poverty and all its hardships and limitations associated with teenage pregnancies, preterm births, single motherhood, or care by other family members resulted in the formulation of the cycle of [socioeconomic] disadvantage and disability. (Chapter on Born Premature: What does it mean?)

INTELLECTUAL DISABILITY AND ECONOMIC SECURITY

The cost of care for children with IDD is substantial and a combination of limited insurance reimbursement and limited public resources can put a significant economic burden on a family. This is further complicated by the reality that children with IDD may be ill more often and need more care than their typical brothers and sisters. As a result, the ability of a parent to maintain employment may be compromised. For a two-parent family, one parent may have to stop working to attend to the needs of the child resulting in a reduction in the family income and potentially tipping the scales into poverty. This is even more difficult for the single-parent family who may already be living on the borderline of poverty. If a single parent has to work then day care is required, which is also costly, or another family member can be recruited. While this is workable in a multigenerational extended family situation, it is not feasible in the nuclear family situation that is more common in the US and other western countries. Thus, not only is poverty – or the state of being poor – associated with an increase likelihood of IDD, but the presence of IDD may precipitate a situation of poverty. For adults with IDD who are unable to earn a living, there is a dependence on family or public funding for support and they are de facto poor (30).

COSTS OF CARE RELATED TO SOCIAL DETERMINANTS OF HEALTH AND HEALTH DISPARITIES

Costs of care are not only borne by the families, the whole of society is involved. Costs of healthcare in the US have soared out of proportion to the benefits. In fact, the US falls behind a number of countries in terms of infant mortality (1) and overall life expectancy despite already high and rising expenditures in healthcare. The reason is that there is major problem of heath disparities related to SDH in the US. As we have reviewed, young women who grow up in poverty are more likely to become pregnant and give birth to premature infants who require neonatal intensive care and are more likely to have CP. The costs of neonatal care are great and the costs of care for children with CP are great, which add to the overall burden of healthcare costs. A simple consideration for prevention of even one pregnancy can result in a significant cost saving in neonatal intensive care as well as in the care needed by the child with CP – a worthwhile return on investment.

CYCLE OF ENVIRONMENTAL HEALTH DISPARITIES

Children who grow up in circumstances of social and economic disadvantage are more likely to be exposed to adverse environmental factors and are more vulnerable to the effects of the environmental factors that affect their health and development as well as their health as adults and chances of success.

These environmental factors then result in limitations in function and, because the additional factors of limited education and the consequent limitations on potential employment and income, residential options are limited and self-determination toward self-fulfillment is significantly compromised. Furthermore, the hormonal changes of the chronic and toxic stress may result in alterations of the immune system and hence, tendency to infectious illnesses and chronic inflammation is increased. These stress responses may also result in disorders that emerge in adulthood such as obesity, diabetes, hypertension, and cerebrovascular accidents (24). Thus, as a consequence of SDH and health disparities, these children, adolescents and adults become part of a self-perpetuating cycle – a cycle of environmental health disparities. (See Chapter on Born Premature: What does it mean?)

This cycle enables the conceptualization not only of specific determinants of health, but also of where interventions can be directed to Break the Cycle and improve the outcome not only for one person but for subsequent generations and ultimately for society as a whole (see figure 3) Although it is gravely daunting and seemingly insurmountable to take on this challenge that requires incalculable costs and unimaginable organization, the world body, in the UN and WHO have set guild lines in their articulation of SDH, and global strategies and goals with their MDG, with frequent documentation of changes and positive differences that have resulted from action taken by various governmental and non-governmental bodies in the quest for global health equity. But we still have a long way to go and there is much to do. Although local, national and international efforts are directed at this in many ways; not

                    I Leslie Rubin

only directly with a focus on health and healthcare, but also on nutrition, agriculture, education, social systems as well as many other creative strategies like the simple project of providing nets for beds to reduce the likelihood of being bitten by mosquitoes and contracting malaria and reduce the associated morbidity and mortality.

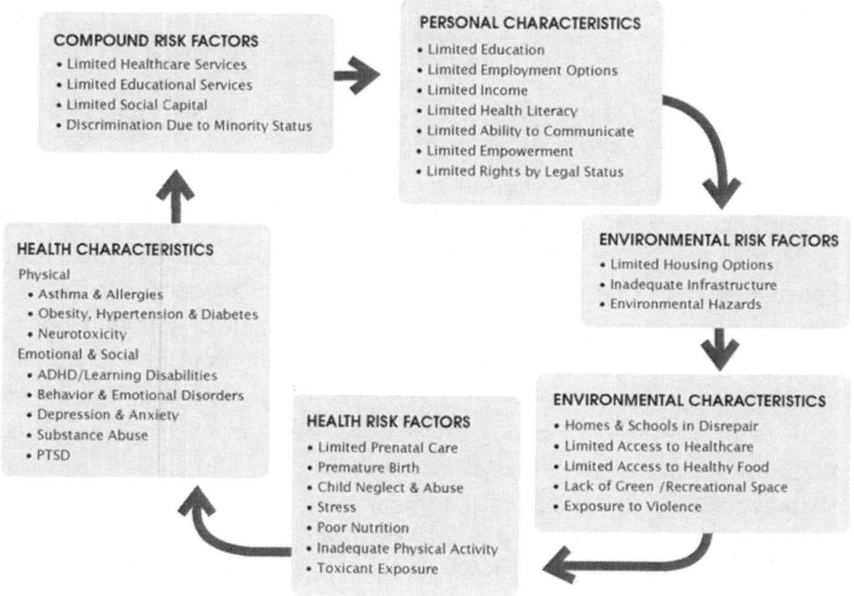

Figure 3. Cycle of environmental health disparities.

Our challenge as a society is to continue to develop strategies to break this cycle of health disparities by any means. Although it is not not possible to change the whole world directly, but with every little effort directed at one child, one person, one condition or one situation at a time, we can all make a big difference. There is a saying that "whoever saves a life, it is considered as if he saved an entire world" (31).

BREAK THE CYCLE PROJECTS

'Break the cycle' is a not uncommon refrain, however, in this context it refers specifically to the cycle of environmental health disparities, the reduction in

SDH conditions and to a potential improvement for the lives of children and their families with an optimistic view to changing the world one project at a time.

In 2004, the author and colleagues (32-35) launched a simple, inexpensive project to create strategies to break the cycle by raising awareness and cultivating leadership in the next generation of professionals. "Break the cycle" is an annual program that selects students from different universities and different academic disciplines to develop projects that will reduce health disparities. The program provides students with a platform for scientific projects that will look at reducing health disparities, and mentors the students in the development and presentation of their projects. The anticipated outcome is that these students will take the lessons they learned in their projects and build on them to become our future leaders in shaping the world for the better.

Program details

The students are required to secure a mentor in their university to guide and support them in their project and submit a formal application. The set of applications for any given year are reviewed for appropriateness, for quality and for the likelihood of success with a set of about ten projects chosen for any given year. Clear guidelines and requirements are provided. The set of students and their mentors then 'meet' together via conference call on a monthly basis for the duration of the project periods. During these meetings, each student presents an update of his or her project which is discussed and commented.

The goal of the program is for the students to present their completed projects at a conference at the end of the project period, and then to write up their projects for publication in a peer reviewed journal. To date, as of the time of writing, there have been nine such annual programs with over 80 students participating from more than 20 different universities and disciplines in the continental US and from Latin America, with a publication of six monographs in international journals and a series of four themed books. The students have been surveyed and the unpublished results show that they benefitted from their participation in the project in many different ways: that they learned about environmental health disparities, and that they continue to be involved in the field of their interest. In addition, they have benefited from being involved in a presentation at an international conference, had a publication and had the opportunity to interact with peers and mentors from other disciplines, other universities and other parts of the world. Examples of the projects include: health impacts of poverty, impact of the built environment on a variety of medical and developmental condition, environmental toxins, air pollution, smoking, substance abuse, depression, crime and violence, maternal and child health, promoting healthy behaviors among adolescents, HIV/AIDS, food, food aid to developing countries, vaccines in developing countries, urban and community gardens, schools and education, laws and international treaties, environmental justice, family structure, the media and a host of other projects that deal with poverty and disenfranchisement (32-35).

CONCLUSION

Adverse social and economic factors affect the health, growth and development of children and can result in chronic health conditions such a hypertension, diabetes and neurodevelopmental disorders (24,25). The factors involved at a macro level in different countries as well as within countries, as well as the micro levels that are reflected in the lives of individuals and their families, are challenging and may be difficult to remedy, but success stories abound in the pursuit of health equity. In this chapter, the connections between SHD and health disparities have been explored and examples of local and global efforts to break the cycle have been offered. The ultimate success of achieving health equity however, it is for as many people as possible to engage in this effort in as many different and creative small and large ways. Remember: It is not incumbent upon you to complete the task, but neither are you free to absolve yourself from undertaking it (36).

ACKNOWLEDGMENTS

This paper is an adapted and revised version of an earlier publication: Rubin IL.

Social determinants of health. In: Rubin IL, Merrick J, Greydanus DE, Patel DR, eds. Rubin and Crocker 3rd edition: Health care for people with intellectual and developmental disabilities across the lifespan. Dordrecht: Springer, 2014

REFERENCES

[1] CIA. The World Factbook: Infant mortality rate. URL: https://www.cia.gov/library/publications/the-world-factbook/rankorder/2091rank.html

[2] Murthy RS, Lakshminarayana R. Mental health consequences of war: A brief review of research findings. World Psychiatry 2006;5(1):25–30.

[3] Brown MJ, McWeeney G, Kim R, Tahirukaj A, Bulat P, Syla S, et al. Lead poisoning among internally displaced Roma, Ashkali and Egyptian children in the United Nations-Administered Province of Kosovo. Eur J Public Health 2010;20(3):288-92.

[4] Commission on Social Determinants of Health (CSDH). Closing the gap in a generation: Health equity through action on the social determinants of health. Final report of the Commission on Social Determinants of Health. Geneva: World Health Organization, 2008.

[5] Millenium goals. URL: http://www.un.org/millenniumgoals/

[6] Boo K. Behind the beautiful forevers. New York: Random House, 2012.

[7] Slum population in India. URL: http://www.indiaonlinepages.com/population/slum-population-in-india.html

[8] Dooyema CA, Neri A, Lo YC, Durant J, Dargan PI, Swarthout T, et al. Outbreak of fatal childhood lead poisoning related to artisanal gold mining in northwestern Nigeria, 2010. Environ Health Perspect 2012;120 (4):601-7.

[9] Spiegel SJ, Veiga MM. Building capacity in small-scale mining communities: Health, ecosystem sustainability and the Global Mercury Project. Eco Health 2005;2(4):1-10

[10] World Health Organization. Exposure to lead: A major public health concern. Geneva: WHO, 2010.

[11] US Department of Health and Human Services, Healthy People 2020, Draft. Washington, DC: US Government Printing Office, 2009.

[12] Rubin IL, Nodvin JT, Geller RJ, Teague WG, Holzclaw BL, Felner EI. Environmental health disparities and social impact of industrial pollution in a community – the model of Anniston, AL. Pediatr Clin North Am 2007;54:375-98.

[13] Etzel RA, Balk SJ. Pediatric environmental health, 3rd ed. Elk Grove, IL: AAP, 2012:13-25.

[14] Frederick CB., Snellman K, Putnam RD, Increasing socioeconomic disparities in adolescent obesity. PNAS 2014;111(4):1338–42.

[15] Beck AF, Huang B, Simmons JM, Moncrief T, Sauers HS, Chen C, et al. Role of financial and social hardships in asthma racial disparities. Pediatrics 2014;133(3):431-9.

[16] Akinbami LJ, Moorman JE, Bailey C, Zahran HS, King M, Johnson CA, Liu X. Trends in asthma prevalence, health care use, and mortality in the United States, 2001–2010. NCHS Data Brief 2012;94:1-8.

[17] Gindi RM, Cohen RA, Kirzinger WK. Emergency room use among adults aged 18–64: Early release of estimates from the National Health Interview Survey, January–

June 2011. National Center for Health Statistics, 2012. URL: http://www.cdc.gov/nchs/nhis/releases.htm.

[18]   Chapman C, Laird J, Ifill N, Kewal Ramani A. Trends in high school dropout and completion rates in the United States, 1972–2009. Compendium report. Washington, DC: US Department of Education, NCES, 2011.

[19]   Bania M. Gang violence among youth and young adults: (Dis)affiliation and the potential for prevention. IPC Rev 2009;3:89–116.

[20]   Finer LB, Zolna MR Unintended pregnancy in the United States: Incidence and disparities, 2006. Contraception 2011;84(5)478-85.

[21]   HIV prevention in the United States: Expanding the impact. URL:http://www.cdc.gov/nchhstp/newsroom/HIVFactSheets/Epidemic/Factors.htm

[22]   Gilbert W, Jandial D, Field N, Bigelow P, Danielsen B Birth outcomes in teenage pregnancies. J Matern Fetal Neonat Med 2004;16(5) 265-70.

[23]   Rubin IL, Geller RJ, Nodvin J, Ace K, Merrick J. Break the cycle to improve health and developmental outcomes for all children. Int J Child Adolesc Health 2009;2:265-72.

[24]   Shonkoff JP, Garner AS. Committee on Psychosocial Aspects of Child and Family Health; Committee on Early Childhood, Adoption, and Dependent Care; Section on Developmental and Behavioral Pediatrics. The lifelong effects of early childhood adversity and toxic stress. Pediatrics 2012;129(1):e232-46.

[25]   Wood D. Effect of child and family poverty on child health in the United States. Pediatrics 2003;112(3):707.

[26]   Mani A, Mullainathan S, Shafir E, Zhao J. Poverty impedes cognitive function. Science 2013;341(6149):976-80.

[27]   Mandell DS, Wiggins LD, Carpenter LA, Daniels J, DiGuiseppi C, Durkin MS, et al. Racial/ethnic disparities in the identification of children with autism spectrum disorders. Am J Public Health 2009;99(3):493–8.

[28]   Zito JM, Safer DJ, Sai D, Gardner JF, Thomas D, Coombes P, et al. Psychotropic medication patterns among youth in foster care. Pediatrics 2008;121(1):e157-63.

[29]   Maenner MJ, Benedict RE, Arneson CL, Yeargin-Allsopp M, Wingate MS, Kirby RS, et al Children with cerebral palsy: racial disparities in functional limitations. Epidemiology 2012;23(1):35-43.

[30]   Emerson E. Poverty and people with intellectual disabilities. Ment Retard Dev Disabil Res Rev 2007;13(2):107–13.

[31]   Mishnah Sanhedrin 4:9; Babylonian Talmud Tractate Sanhedrin 37a.

[32]   Rubin IL, Merrick J, eds. Environmental health: Home school and community. New York: Nova Science, 2013.

[33]   Rubin IL, Merrick J, eds. Environmental health disparities in children: Asthma, obesity and food. New York: Nova Science, 2013.

[34]   Rubin IL, Merrick J,eds. Child health and human development: Social, economic and environmental factors. New York: Nova Science, 2013.

[35]   Rubin IL, Merrick J, eds. Break the cycle of environmental health disparities: Maternal and child health aspects. New York: Nova Science, 2013.

[36]   Pirke Avot; Chapter 2: mishna 16.

SECTION TWO: ACKNOWLEDGEMENTS

In: Born into this World: Health Issues   ISBN: 978-1-63321-667-9
Editors: D. E. Greydanus, A. N. Feinberg et al.   © 2014 Nova Science Publishers, Inc.

Chapter 10

ABOUT THE EDITORS

Donald E Greydanus, MD, Dr. HC (Athens), FAAP, FSAM (Emeritus), FIAP (HON) is Professor and Founding Chair of the Department of Pediatric and Adolescent Medicine, as well as Pediatrics Program Director at the Western Michigan University Homer Stryker MD School of Medicine (WMED), Kalamazoo, Michigan, USA. He is also Professor of Pediatrics and Human Development at Michigan State University College of Human Medicine (East Lansing, Michigan, USA) as well as Clinical Professor of Pediatrics at MSU College of Osteopathic Medicine in East Lansing, Michigan, USA. Received the 1995 American Academy of Pediatrics' Adele D. Hofmann Award for "Distinguished Contributions in Adolescent Health", the 2000 Mayo Clinic Pediatrics Honored Alumnus Award for "National Contributions to the field of Pediatrics," and the 2003 William B Weil, Jr., MD Endowed Distinguished Pediatric Faculty Award from Michigan State University College of Medicine for "National and international recognition as well as exemplary scholarship in pediatrics." Received the 2004 Charles R Drew School of Medicine (Los Angeles, CA) Stellar Award for contributions to pediatric resident education and awarded an honorary membership in the Indian Academy of Pediatrics—an honor granted to only a few pediatricians outside of India. Was the 2007-2010 Visiting Professor of Pediatrics at Athens University, Athens, Greece and received the Michigan State University College of Human Medicine Outstanding Community Faculty Award in 2008. In 2010 he received the title of Doctor Honoris Causa from the University of Athens (Greece) as a "distinguished scientist who through outstanding work has bestowed praise and credit on the field of adolescent medicine (Ephebiatrics)." In 2010 he received the Outstanding Achievement in Adolescent Medicine Award from the Society for Adolescent Medicine "as a leading force in the field of adolescent medicine and health." Past Chair of the National Conference and

Exhibition Planning Group (Committee on Scientific Meetings) of the American Academy of Pediatrics and member of the Pediatric Academic Societies' (SPR/PAS) Planning Committee (1998 to Present). In 2011 elected to The Alpha Omega Alpha Honor Society (Faculty member) at Michigan State University College of Human Medicine, East Lansing, Michigan. Former member of the Appeals Committee for the Pediatrics' Residency Review Committee (RRC) of the Accreditation Council for Graduate Medical Education (Chicago, IL) in both adolescent medicine and general pediatrics. Numerous publications in adolescent health and lectureships in many countries on adolescent health. E-mail: donald.greydanus@med.wmich.edu

Arthur N Feinberg, MD, FAAP is professor of Pediatrics and Adolescent Medicine at the Western Michigan University in Kalamazoo, Michigan, United States. He is also Professor of Pediatrics at the Michigan State University College of Human Medicine, Department of Pediatrics and Human Development, East Lansing, Michigan, as well as Clinical Professor of Pediatrics at the Michigan State University College of Osteopathic Medicine. He attended the Albert Einstein College of Medicine at the Yeshiva University in New York and completed pediatric internship and residency at Montefiore Hospital and Medical Center in New York. After serving two years in the US Navy he entered private practice in Kalamazoo in 1975. His strong interest in teaching led him to join the residency program in Kalamazoo in 1993. He has been recipient of six teaching awards since joining the faculty. His research interests have included newborn topics such as hospital discharge and circumcision and have led to several original publications and numerous book chapters. He has been co-editor of three textbooks. E-mail: arthur.feinberg@med.wmich.edu

Joav Merrick, MD, MMedSci, DMSc, is professor of pediatrics, child health and human development, Division of Pediatrics, Hadassah Hebrew University Medical Center, Mt Scopus Campus, Jerusalem, Israel and Kentucky Children's Hospital, University of Kentucky, Lexington, Kentucky United States and professor of public health at the Center for Healthy Development, School of Public Health, Georgia State University, Atlanta, United States, the medical director of the Health Services, Division for Intellectual and Developmental Disabilities, Ministry of Social Affairs and Social Services, Jerusalem, the founder and director of the National Institute of Child Health and Human Development in Israel. Numerous publications in the field of pediatrics, child health and human development, rehabilitation, intellectual disability, disability, health, welfare, abuse, advocacy, quality of life and prevention. Received the Peter Sabroe Child Award for outstanding work on behalf of Danish Children in 1985 and the International LEGO-Prize ("The Children's Nobel Prize") for an extraordinary contribution towards improvement in child welfare and well-being in 1987. E-mail: jmerrick@zahav.net.il

In: Born into this World: Health Issues
Editors: D. E. Greydanus, A. N. Feinberg et al.

ISBN: 978-1-63321-667-9
© 2014 Nova Science Publishers, Inc.

Chapter 11

ABOUT THE DEPARTMENT OF PEDIATRIC AND ADOLESCENT MEDICINE, WESTERN MICHIGAN UNIVERSITY HOMER STRYKER MD SCHOOL OF MEDICINE (WMED), KALAMAZOO, MICHIGAN USA

MISSION AND SERVICE

The Western Michigan University Homer Stryker MD School of Medicine was started in 2012 and its first class of medical students began in 2014. The Department of Pediatric and Adolescent Medicine has a pediatric residency program which is accredited by the Accreditation Council for Graduate Medical Education (ACGME) in Chicago, Illinois, USA and the current residency program in Pediatrics started in 1990.

The WMED Department of Pediatric and Adolescent Medicine has a commitment to a comprehensive approach to the health and development of the child, adolescent, and the family. The Department has a blend of academic general pediatricians and pediatric specialists. Our Pediatric Clinic team provides a broad spectrum of general well and sick child care (birth through 18 years) including immunizations, monitoring general physical and emotional growth, motor skill development, sports medicine (including participation evaluations and evaluation of common sports injuries), child abuse evaluations, and psychosocial or behavioral assessment. WMED Pediatrics believes in immunizations as a protection against preventative disease processes. Our Pediatrics Clinic is undergoing a transformation to a patient-centered medical home (PCMH). A patient-centered medical home is a way to deliver coordinated and comprehensive primary care to our infants, children, adolescents and young adults. It is a partnership between individuals and families within a health care setting, which allows for a more efficient use of resources and time to improve the quality of outcomes for all involved through care provided by a continuity care team.

RESEARCH ACTIVITIES

The Department has a variety of research projects in adolescent medicine, neurobehavioral pediatrics, adolescent gynecology, pediatric diabetes mellitus, asthma, and cystic fibrosis. The WMED Department of Pediatric and Adolescent Medicine has published a number of medical textbooks: Essential adolescent medicine (McGraw-Hill Medical Publishers), The pediatric diagnostic examination (McGraw-Hill), Pediatric and adolescent psychopharmacology (Cambridge University Press), Behavioral pediatrics, 2nd edition (iUniverse Publishers in New York and Lincoln, Nebraska), Behavioral pediatrics 3rd edition (New York: Nova Biomedical Books); 4th Edition: In press. Pediatric practice: Sports medicine (McGraw-Hill), Handbook of clinical pediatrics (Singapore: World Scientific), Neurodevelopmental disabilities: Clinical care for children and young adults (Dordrecht: Springer), Adolescent medicine: Pharmacotherapeutics in medical disorders (Berlin/Boston: De Gruyter), Adolescent medicine: Pharmacotherapeutics in general, mental, and sexual health (Berlin/Boston: De Gruyter), Pediatric psychodermatology (Berlin/Boston: De Gruyter), Substance abuse in adolescents and young adults: A manual for pediatric and primary care clinicians (Berlin/Boston: De Gruyter), and tropical pediatrics (New York: Nova); Second edition in press.

The Department has edited a number of journal issues published by Elsevier Publishers covering pulmonology (State of the Art Reviews: Adolescent Medicine—AM:STARS), genetic disorders in adolescents (AM:STARS), neurologic/neurodevelopmental disorders (AM:STARS), behavioral pediatrics (Pediatric Clinics of North America), pediatric psychopharmacology in the 21st century (Pediatric Clinic of North America), nephrologic disorders in adolescents (AM:STARS), college health (Pediatric Clinics of North America), adolescent medicine (Primary Care: Clinics in Office Practice), behavioral pediatrics in children and adolescents (Primary Care: Clinics in Office Practice), adolescents and sports (Pediatric Clinics of North America), and developmental disabilities (Pediatric Clinics of North

America). The Department has also edited a journal issue on musculoskeletal disorders in children and adolescents for the American Academy of Pediatrics' AM:STARs; in April of 2013 a Subspecialty Update issue was published in AM:STARs.

The department has developed academic ties with a variety of international medical centers and organizations, including the Queen Elizabeth Hospital in Hong Kong, Indian Academy of Pediatrics (New Delhi, India), the University of Athens Children's Hospital (First and Second Departments of Paediatrics) in Athens, Greece and the National Institute of Child Health and Human Development in Jerusalem, Israel.

CONTACT

Professor Donald E Greydanus, MD and Professor Dilip R. Patel, MD
Department of Pediatric and Adolescent Medicine, Western Michigan
University Homer Stryker MD School of Medicine, 1000 Oakland Drive,
D48G, Kalamazoo, MI 49008-1284, United States,
E-mail: Donald.greydanus@med.wmich.edu and dilip.Patel@med.wmich.edu,
Website: http://www.med.wmich.edu

In: Born into this World: Health Issues
Editors: D. E. Greydanus, A. N. Feinberg et al.

ISBN: 978-1-63321-667-9
© 2014 Nova Science Publishers, Inc.

Chapter 12

ABOUT THE NATIONAL INSTITUTE OF CHILD HEALTH AND HUMAN DEVELOPMENT IN ISRAEL

The National Institute of Child Health and Human Development (NICHD) in Israel was established in 1998 as a virtual institute under the auspices of the Medical Director, Ministry of Social Affairs and Social Services in order to function as the research arm for the Office of the Medical Director. In 1998 the National Council for Child Health and Pediatrics, Ministry of Health and in 1999 the Director General and Deputy Director General of the Ministry of Health endorsed the establishment of the NICHD.

MISSION

The mission of a National Institute for Child Health and Human Development in Israel is to provide an academic focal point for the scholarly interdisciplinary study of child life, health, public health, welfare, disability, rehabilitation, intellectual disability and related aspects of human development. This mission includes research, teaching, clinical work, information and public service activities in the field of child health and human development.

SERVICE AND ACADEMIC ACTIVITIES

Over the years many activities became focused in the south of Israel due to collaboration with various professionals at the Faculty of Health Sciences (FOHS) at the Ben Gurion University of the Negev (BGU). Since 2000 an affiliation with the Zusman Child Development Center at the Pediatric Division of Soroka University Medical Center has resulted in collaboration around the establishment of the Down Syndrome Clinic at that center. In 2002 a full course on "Disability" was established at the Recanati School for Allied Professions in the Community, FOHS, BGU and in 2005 collaboration was started with the Primary Care Unit of the faculty and disability became part of the master of public health course on "Children and society". In the academic year 2005-2006 a one semester course on "Aging with disability" was started as part of the master of science program in gerontology in our collaboration with the Center for Multidisciplinary Research in Aging. In 2010 collaborations with the Division of Pediatrics, Hadassah Hebrew University Medical Center, Jerusalem, Israel around the National Down Syndrome Center and teaching students and residents about intellectual and developmental disabilities as part of their training at this campus.

RESEARCH ACTIVITIES

The affiliated staff have over the years published work from projects and research activities in this national and international collaboration. In the year 2000 the International Journal of Adolescent Medicine and Health and in 2005 the International Journal on Disability and Human Development of De Gruyter Publishing House (Berlin and New York) were affiliated with the National Institute of Child Health and Human Development. From 2008 also the International Journal of Child Health and Human Development (Nova Science, New York), the International Journal of Child and Adolescent Health (Nova Science) and the Journal of Pain Management (Nova Science) affiliated and from 2009 the International Public Health Journal (Nova Science) and Journal of Alternative Medicine Research (Nova Science). All peer-reviewed international journals.

NATIONAL COLLABORATIONS

Nationally the NICHD works in collaboration with the Faculty of Health Sciences, Ben Gurion University of the Negev; Department of Physical Therapy, Sackler School of Medicine, Tel Aviv University; Autism Center, Assaf HaRofeh Medical Center; National Rett and PKU Centers at Chaim Sheba Medical Center, Tel HaShomer; Department of Physiotherapy, Haifa University; Department of Education, Bar Ilan University, Ramat Gan, Faculty of Social Sciences and Health Sciences; College of Judea and Samaria in Ariel and in 2011 affiliation with Center for Pediatric Chronic Diseases and National Center for Down Syndrome, Department of Pediatrics, Hadassah Hebrew University Medical Center, Mount Scopus Campus, Jerusalem.

INTERNATIONAL COLLABORATIONS

Internationally with the Department of Disability and Human Development, College of Applied Health Sciences, University of Illinois at Chicago; Strong Center for Developmental Disabilities, Golisano Children's Hospital at Strong, University of Rochester School of Medicine and Dentistry, New York; Centre on Intellectual Disabilities, University of Albany, New York; Centre for Chronic Disease Prevention and Control, Health Canada, Ottawa; Chandler Medical Center and Children's Hospital, Kentucky Children's Hospital, Section of Adolescent Medicine, University of Kentucky, Lexington; Chronic Disease Prevention and Control Research Center, Baylor College of Medicine, Houston, Texas; Division of Neuroscience, Department of Psychiatry, Columbia University, New York; Institute for the Study of Disadvantage and Disability, Atlanta; Center for Autism and Related Disorders, Department Psychiatry, Children's Hospital Boston, Boston; Department of Paediatrics, Child Health and Adolescent Medicine, Children's Hospital at Westmead, Westmead, Australia; International Centre for the Study of Occupational and Mental Health, Düsseldorf, Germany; Centre for Advanced Studies in Nursing, Department of General Practice and Primary Care, University of Aberdeen, Aberdeen, United Kingdom; Quality of Life Research Center, Copenhagen, Denmark; Nordic School of Public Health, Gottenburg, Sweden, Scandinavian Institute of Quality of Working Life, Oslo, Norway; The Department of Applied Social Sciences (APSS) of The Hong Kong Polytechnic University Hong Kong.

TARGETS

Our focus is on research, international collaborations, clinical work, teaching and policy in health, disability and human development and to establish the NICHD as a permanent institute at one of the residential care centers for persons with intellectual disability in Israel in order to conduct model research and together with the four university schools of public health/medicine in Israel establish a national master and doctoral program in disability and human development at the institute to secure the next generation of professionals working in this often non-prestigious/low-status field of work.

CONTACT

Joav Merrick, MD, MMedSci, DMSc
Professor of Pediatrics, Child Health and Human Development
Medical Director, Health Services, Division for Intellectual and
Developmental Disabilities, Ministry of Social Affairs and Social Services,
POB 1260, IL-91012 Jerusalem, Israel.
E-mail: jmerrick@zahav.net.il

In: Born into this World: Health Issues   ISBN: 978-1-63321-667-9
Editors: D. E. Greydanus, A. N. Feinberg et al.   © 2014 Nova Science Publishers, Inc.

Chapter 13

ABOUT THE BOOK SERIES "PEDIATRICS, CHILD AND ADOLESCENT HEALTH"

Pediatrics, child and adolescent health is a book series with publications from a multidisciplinary group of researchers, practitioners and clinicians for an international professional forum interested in the broad spectrum of pediatric medicine, child health, adolescent health and human development.

- Merrick J, ed. Child and adolescent health yearbook 2011. New York: Nova Science, 2012.
- Merrick J, ed. Child and adolescent health yearbook 2012. New York: Nova Science, 2012.
- Roach RR, Greydanus DE, Patel DR, Homnick DN, Merrick J, eds. Tropical pediatrics: A public health concern of international proportions. New York: Nova Science, 2012.
- Merrick J, ed. Child health and human development yearbook 2011. New York: Nova Science, 2012.
- Merrick J, ed. Child health and human development yearbook 2012. New York: Nova Science, 2012.
- Shek DTL, Sun RCF, Merrick J, eds. Developmental issues in Chinese adolescents. New York: Nova Science, 2012.
- Shek DTL, Sun RCF, Merrick J, eds. Positive youth development: Theory, research and application. New York: Nova Science, 2012.
- Zachor DA, Merrick J, eds. Understanding autism spectrum disorder: Current research aspects. New York: Nova Science, 2012.

- Ma HK, Shek DTL, Merrick J, eds. Positive youth development: A new school curriculum to tackle adolescent developmental issues. New York: Nova Science, 2012.
- Wood D, Reiss JG, Ferris ME, Edwards LR, Merrick J, eds. Transition from pediatric to adult medical care. New York: Nova Science, 2012.
- Isenberg Y. Guidelines for the healthy integration of the ill child in the educational system: Experience from Israel. New York: Nova Science, 2013.
- Shek DTL, Sun RCF, Merrick J, eds. Chinese adolescent development: Economic disadvantages, parents and intrapersonal development. New York: Nova Science, 2013.
- Shek DTL, Sun RCF, Merrick J, eds. University and college students: Health and development issues for the leaders of tomorrow. New York: Nova Science, 2013.
- Shek DTL, Sun RCF, Merrick J, eds. Adolescence and behavior issues in a Chinese context. New York: Nova Science, 2013.
- Sun J, Buys N, Merrick J, eds. Advances in preterm infant research. New York: Nova Science, 2013.
- Tsitsika A, Janikian M, Greydanus DE, Omar HA, Merrick J, eds. Internet addiction: A public health concern in adolescence. New York: Nova Science, 2013.
- Shek DTL, Lee TY, Merrick J, eds. Promotion of holistic development of young people in Hong Kong. New York: Nova Science, 2013.
- Shek DTL, Ma C, Lu Y, Merrick J, eds. Human developmental research: Experience from research in Hong Kong. New York: Nova Science, 2013.
- Merrick J, ed. Chronic disease and disability in childhood. New York: Nova Science, 2013.
- Rubin IL, Merrick J, eds. Break the cycle of environmental health disparities: Maternal and child health aspects. New York: Nova Science, 2013.
- Rubin IL, Merrick J, eds. Environmental health disparities in children: Asthma, obesity and food. New York: Nova Science, 2013.
- Rubin IL, Merrick J, eds. Environmental health: Home, school and community. New York: Nova Science, 2013.

- Rubin IL, Merrick J, eds. Child health and human development: Social, economic and environmental factors. New York: Nova Science, 2013.
- Merrick J, Kandel I, Omar HA, eds. Children, violence and bullying: International perspectives. New York: Nova Science, 2013.
- Omar HA, Bowling CH, Merrick J, eds. Playing with fire: Children, adolescents and firesetting. New York: Nova Science, 2013.
- Merrick J, Tenenbaum A, Omar HA, eds. School, adolescence and health issues. New York: Nova Science, 2013.
- Merrick J, Tenenbaum A, Omar Ha, eds. Adolescence and sexuality: International perspectives. New York: Nova Science, 2014.
- Diamond G, Arbel E. Adoption: The search for a new parenthood. New York: Nova Science, 2014.
- Taylor MF, Pooley JA, Merrick J, eds. Adolescence: Places and spaces. New York: Nova Science, 2014.

Contact

Professor Joav Merrick, MD, MMedSci, DMSc
Medical Director, Medical Services
Division for Intellectual and Developmental Disabilities
Ministry of Social Affairs and Social Services
POBox 1260, IL-91012 Jerusalem, Israel
E-mail: jmerrick@zahav.net.il

SECTION THREE: INDEX

INDEX

#

20th century, 5, 10, 107, 162
21st century, 7, 10, 11, 161, 182

A

Abraham, 6, 13
abuse, 31, 61, 116, 155, 165, 166, 179, 182
academic performance, 163
access, 60, 76, 91, 94, 95, 117, 140, 149,
    160, 162, 163, 164
accountability, 94
accounting, 124, 138
achalasia, 55
acid, 56, 85, 86, 87, 98, 139
acidosis, 24, 30, 79
acrocyanosis, 29, 54
ACTH, 62
acute lymphoblastic leukemia, 108
acute stress, 148
adaptability, 50
adaptation, 73, 155
adduction, 44
ADHD, 123, 124, 130, 166
adhesions, 136, 138
adipose, 71
adipose tissue, 71
adjustment, 56
adolescent development, 190

adolescents, 169, 172, 182, 189, 191
adrenal gland(s), 39
adrenaline, 148
adrenogenital syndrome, 57
adulthood, 128, 130, 144, 165, 166, 169
adults, 107, 124, 137, 158, 163, 165, 168,
    169, 173, 182
advancement(s), 9, 83
adverse effects, 152
advocacy, 96, 179
affluence, 161
Afghanistan, 158
Africa, 122, 161
African-American, 88, 155
age, 19, 20, 26, 28, 29, 33, 34, 48, 49, 50,
    71, 74, 77, 81, 84, 91, 96, 99, 100, 116,
    118, 130, 132, 158, 160, 161, 164
agencies, 152
aggregation, 145
agriculture, 170
AIDS, 164
air quality, 164
airways, 10
albumin, 79
alcohol use, 116, 149
alertness, 28, 43
algorithm, 73, 75, 105, 106
alternative treatments, 139
alters, 120, 147
alveoli, 104, 108, 118
amblyopia, 33

American Heart Association, 101, 102, 111
amino, 26, 86
amino acid(s), 26, 86
aminoglycosides, 99
ammonia, 6
amniotic fluid, 27, 28, 35, 55, 71, 107
amputation, 40, 138
anabolic steroids, 24
anastomosis, 138
anatomy, 32, 39, 40
androgen(s), 39, 40, 62
anemia, 21, 23, 57, 85, 110
anencephaly, 44
angulation, 42, 138
aniridia, 33
annular pancreas, 55
antenatal departments, 4
antibiotic, 51, 76, 77, 138
antibiotic ointment, 138
antibody, 21, 73
antisocial behavior, 125
anus, 40, 55
anxiety, 88, 91, 95, 97, 144, 148, 153
aorta, 103
aortic stenosis, 24, 53
apnea, 6, 19, 20, 24, 28, 73, 105, 119
appetite, 149
architect, 12
armed conflict, 158
arousal, 27
arrest, 65, 164
arrhythmias, 26
arterial blood gas, 71
artery(s), 38, 103
arterioles, 104
arthrogryposis, 40
articulation, 169
ascites, 38
aseptic, 10
Asia, 122, 161
asphyxia, 15, 29, 79, 101, 102, 122, 129
aspiration, 35, 52, 71
assessment, 19, 20, 27, 29, 31, 43, 48, 61,
    77, 94, 105, 151, 155
assessment tools, 94

asthma, 153, 164, 173, 182
asymmetry, 44, 52
asymptomatic, 51, 54, 73, 92
atelectasis, 13
athetosis, 43
atmosphere, 71, 127
atrophy, 36
attitudes, 166
auscultation, 20, 31, 36
autism, 123, 130, 166, 174, 189
autoimmune disease, 58
autoimmunity, 58
autonomy, 94
autosomal dominant, 57, 59
autosomal recessive, 38, 59
average costs, 126
awareness, 119, 120, 138, 171
axons, 119

B

bacteria, 20, 51, 134
balanitis, 131, 133
balanoposthitis, 132
Balkans, 159
ban, 142
banking, 6
banks, 152
basal ganglia, 120
base, 94
beer, 151
behavioral assessment, 181
behaviors, 117, 144, 148, 149, 164, 172
beneficiaries, 91, 92
benefits, 71, 83, 85, 91, 94, 99, 123, 132,
    134, 136, 140, 168
benign, 27, 31, 32, 33, 34, 38, 40, 52, 53,
    54, 56, 57, 92
bias, 92, 95
bicarbonate, 109
bile, 55, 58, 59
bile duct, 59
biliary atresia, 59
bilirubin, 23, 49, 57, 58, 63, 77, 79, 118
birth rate, 114

birth weight, ix, 48, 56, 67, 74, 98, 113, 114, 117, 122, 123, 129, 130, 143, 144, 145, 146, 147, 148, 149, 150, 151, 152, 153, 154, 155

births, 5, 67, 70, 74, 114, 115, 116, 117, 122, 123, 124, 128, 158, 168

bleeding, 24, 58, 137, 138, 139

blindness, 24, 33

blood, 6, 8, 14, 23, 27, 39, 49, 51, 52, 55, 57, 58, 61, 62, 63, 71, 72, 73, 76, 77, 89, 90, 92, 95, 98, 102, 103, 104, 105, 108, 109, 110, 118, 148, 149

blood cultures, 63

blood flow, 103, 104, 108, 109, 148, 149

blood group, 58

blood pressure, 71, 103, 105, 118

blood supply, 98

blood transfusion, 14

blood vessels, 103

bloodstream, 58

blueprint, 159

body weight, 4, 71, 163

bone(s), 24, 31

borrowers, 152

bowel, 36, 39, 119

bowel sounds, 39

brachial plexus, 29

bradycardia, 24, 61, 104, 110

brain, 22, 32, 70, 104, 108, 109, 118, 119, 120, 121, 127, 129, 155, 161, 165, 166

brain damage, 161, 165

brain functioning, 119

breakdown, 56, 58

breast feeding, 72, 77, 80

breastfeeding, 4, 49

breathing, 8, 9, 27, 28, 35, 36, 54, 71, 73, 105, 107, 108, 127

breathing rate, 28

bronchial tree, 52, 104

bronchopulmonary dysplasia, 7, 119

brothers, 168

buccal mucosa, 35

bullying, 191

businesses, 152, 163

C

C reactive protein, 51

caesarean section, 10, 52

calcifications, 22

cancer, 23, 133, 134

capillary, 71, 118

carbon, 149

carbon monoxide, 149

carcinoma, 134

cardiac output, 104, 109

cardiologist, 53

cardiovascular system, 118

caregivers, 11, 137

cartilage, 68

casting, 42

cataract, 23

catheter, 35, 55, 107, 138

cattle, 8

causation, 151

CDC, 12, 75, 76, 162, 163

Census, 145, 150

central nervous system (CNS), 40, 114

cephalohematoma, 32, 58

cerebellum, 129

cerebral cortex, 120

cerebral palsy, 5, 12, 115, 121, 122, 123, 129, 174

cerebrospinal fluid, 31, 51

certification, 102

cervical cancer, 134, 141

cervix, 116

cesarean section, 123

challenges, 79, 80, 97, 113, 124, 127, 148, 152

chemical(s), 21, 149, 163

child abuse, 165, 181

Child Behavior Checklist, 124

child development, 160

child labor, 5

child mortality, 111, 159, 161

childcare, 149, 152

childhood, 5, 103, 128, 133, 144, 151, 156, 160, 161, 166, 173, 174, 190

chlamydia, 20, 22

Chlamydia trachomatis, 22
chorea, 95, 97
chorioretinitis, 22
chromatography, 86
chromosomal abnormalities, 37
chylothorax, 25, 52
CIA, 173
cigarette smoking, 149
circulation, 52, 54, 57, 104, 108, 110
circumcision, 131, 132, 133, 134, 135, 136,
    137, 138, 139, 140, 141, 142, 178
cities, 160
citizens, 92, 158, 159, 160, 163
citizenship, 13
classification, 165
clavicle, 29, 61
cleft palate, 23, 35
clinical presentation, 96
clonus, 48
closure, 32, 39, 103, 138, 139, 163
CNN, 142
CNS, 37, 40, 56, 63, 115
CO_2, 54, 108
cocaine, 31
cognition, 92, 119, 161
cognitive defects, 149
cognitive development, 130
cognitive function, 174
cognitive process, 120
collaboration, 15, 186, 187
collagen, 21, 36, 139
collateral, 91, 92
college students, 190
colon, 57
color, 27, 28, 33, 36, 48, 59
coma, 43
commercial, 96
common bile duct, 59
communication, 79
community(s), 84, 93, 115, 116, 124, 128,
    143, 144, 146, 149, 152, 152, 154, 155,
    156, 157, 159, 160, 161, 172, 173, 174,
    190
compensation, 37, 53
complexity, 117, 121, 126, 166

complications, 5, 15, 64, 67, 114, 115, 117,
    118, 122, 124, 131, 133, 136
compounds, 149
compression, 8, 10, 27, 37, 52, 110
conception, 160
conceptualization, 169
conditioning, 164
conduct disorder, 166
conference, 15, 171
confidentiality, 91, 94, 95
conflict, 158, 159
confounding variables, 97
congenital adrenal hyperplasia, 39, 40
congenital heart disease, 37, 50, 53, 54, 57
congenital malformations, 56
conjugated bilirubin, 58, 79
conjugation, 58
conjunctivitis, 22
consciousness, 43
consensus, 10, 15, 97
consent, 97
constipation, 54, 55
consumption, 149
contour, 39
control group, 92, 135
controversial, 131, 141
convention, 131
cooperation, 149
coordination, 31, 149, 152
cornea, 33
corneal opacities, 33
corpus callosum, 23
correlation, 148, 166
cortex, 119, 147
corticosteroid cream, 139
corticosteroids, 139
corticotropin, 148
cortisol, 62, 148, 154
cosmetic, 136
cosmos, 11
cost, 60, 80, 85, 87, 91, 94, 99, 126, 128,
    130, 133, 164, 168, 169
cost effectiveness, 94
cost saving, 169
counsel, 97

counseling, 96, 152
covering, 182
cranial nerve, 35, 43
craniotomy, 10
creatinine, 61, 63
crepitus, 37
Crigler-Najjar syndrome, 59
crown, 66
CRP, 51, 63
crystals, 49
CSF, 31
CT, 61, 62, 63, 127
cues, 153
cultural practices, 157
culture, 76, 146
curriculum, 190
cyanide, 149
cyanosis, 19, 20, 36, 38, 48, 51, 52, 54, 73
cyanotic, 52
cyst, 36, 38, 60, 138
cystic duct, 59
cystic fibrosis, 55, 60, 182
cytomegalovirus, 20, 99

D

dacryocystitis, 32
dacryostenosis, 32
danger, 148, 155
database, 90, 146
deaths, 12, 114, 158
debridement, 138
decay, 154
defects, 23, 24, 32, 33, 35, 58
defibrillation, 10
deficiency, 7, 24, 40, 50, 56, 58, 59, 60, 79, 85, 86, 98, 118
deficit, 123, 130, 166
degenerate, 6
dehydration, 80
Denmark, 187
Department of Education, 174, 187
deposition, 118
depression, 24, 148, 154, 155, 164, 172
depressive symptomatology, 154

deprivation, 150
dermoid cyst, 36
despair, 161
destruction, 137
detachment, 33
detection, 85, 90, 91
developing brain, 122, 124
developing countries, 172
developmental milestones, 93
deviation, 35
diabetes, 21, 23, 25, 29, 50, 72, 89, 90, 116, 117, 151, 163, 169, 172, 182
diaphoresis, 53
diaphragmatic hernia, 23, 36, 38
diarrhea, 6, 75
diet, 73, 84, 85, 92, 96, 149
differential diagnosis, 33, 64
direct bilirubin, 62
direct observation, 36
disability, 84, 85, 97, 113, 123, 125, 129, 144, 145, 151, 153, 162, 166, 168, 179, 185, 186, 188, 190
discharges, 72
discomfort, 39, 43
discrimination, 95, 160, 162
diseases, 5, 35, 60, 108, 132, 135, 159
disorder, 21, 58, 122, 123, 130, 137, 144, 145, 147, 149, 150, 151, 153, 154, 156, 166, 189
dissatisfaction, 148
disseminated intravascular coagulation, 59
distress, 27, 51, 70, 72, 75, 108, 124, 154, 161
distribution, 32, 89, 90, 155, 157, 158, 159
DOC, 62
dopamine, 109
Down syndrome, 33, 36, 53, 58, 61
drainage, 59, 138
drug abuse, 50
drug therapy, 96
drugs, 15, 23, 24, 109, 166
ductus arteriosus, 52, 103, 108
dysplasia, 13, 33, 36, 38, 41

E

ecchymosis, 29
economic disadvantage, 125, 126, 155, 162, 169
economic incentives, 92
economic losses, 95
economic status, 146
economic systems, 159
economics, 93, 160
ecosystem, 173
ectropion, 32
edema, 26, 32, 36, 39, 57
editors, x, 177
educated women, 116
education, 94, 125, 126, 128, 144, 152, 159, 164, 169, 170, 172, 177
educational system, 190
EEG, 56, 63
egg, 4
Egypt, 7, 12
Ehlers-Danlos syndrome, 36
EKG, 61, 62
elaboration, 53
electrocautery, 137, 138
electrolyte, 118
ELISA, 61, 86
emboli, 103
emergency, 164
emotional disabilities, 158
emotional distress, 165
emotional problems, 70
emphysema, 52
employment, 91, 147, 168, 169
encephalitis, 22
encephalopathy, 56, 120, 129, 130
endangered, 8
endocrine, 23, 40, 56, 85, 114
endocrinology, 39
endotracheal intubation, 9, 14
enlargement, 33, 38
environment(s), 71, 79, 80, 97, 121, 126, 143, 144, 145, 146, 147, 148, 149, 150, 151, 152, 153, 154, 155, 156, 166, 172

environmental factors, 115, 157, 163, 166, 169, 174, 191
environmental stress, 152
environmental sustainability, 159
enzyme(s), 27, 58, 72
epidemiology, 129
epidermis, 139
epigenetics, 97
epinephrine, 109, 110, 137
epithelium, 132, 135
equity, 13, 94, 169, 172, 173
erythroblastosis fetalis, 6, 13
estrogen, 62
ethical issues, 83, 84, 99
ethics, 84, 91, 93
ethnic groups, 140
ethnicity, 74, 162
eugenics, 97
Europe, 8, 14, 140
European Parliament, 140
evacuation, 52
evidence, 10, 15, 44, 52, 73, 78, 93, 94, 97, 121, 125, 135, 140, 142, 160
evolution, 84, 99, 102, 140
exchange transfusion, 6, 60
excision, 138
exclusion, 160, 162
exercise, 133
expenditures, 168
exposure, 21, 104, 134, 148, 154, 159, 161
exstrophy, 39
external environment, 120, 149
extracellular matrix, 139
extreme poverty, 159

F

factories, 162, 163
false alarms, 88, 89, 90
false negative, 85, 88, 90, 91, 98
false positive, 85, 88, 90, 91, 98, 99
families, 91, 97, 113, 119, 126, 127, 132, 140, 150, 158, 159, 164, 166, 167, 168, 171, 172, 182
family history, 26

family income, 168
family members, 85, 94, 95, 164, 168
FAS, 149
fasting, 90
fat, 39, 51
fatiguability, 37
fatty acids, 86
fear, 144, 153, 166
female partner, 141
femur, 41
fertility, 116
fetal alcohol syndrome, 35
fetal distress, 116
fetal growth, 23, 30, 116, 149
fetus, 11, 16, 21, 23, 26, 29, 39, 102, 104, 117, 129, 148, 149, 155
fever, 51, 52, 57, 74
fibroblasts, 139
fibrosis, 55
figure-ground, 34
financial, 96, 128, 147, 152, 162, 173
financial resources, 128, 152
flank, 46
flex, 45, 48
flexibility, 80
flight, 44, 148
fluctuations, 118
fluid, 6, 7, 25, 27, 36, 48, 52, 63, 104, 107, 118
fluid management, 6
food, 38, 158, 163, 166, 172, 174, 190
foramen, 103
foramen ovale, 103
force, 41, 177
formation, 52
formula, 92
fractures, 37, 40, 61
fragility, 98
France, 4, 12
freedom, 140, 142
fremitus, 37
frenulum, 138
funding, 168
fusion, 39

G

gallbladder, 38
gangrene, 138
gangs, 164
garbage, 151
gastrointestinal tract, 104, 114
gastroschisis, 23, 24, 38
gender equality, 159
gender equity, 160
general anesthesia, 136, 139
genes, 97
genetic disorders, 182
genetic endowment, 97
genetic information, 95, 97
genetic predisposition, 96
genetic screening, 97
genetic syndromes, 39
genetic testing, 91, 95, 99
genetics, 13, 41, 94
genomics, 83
Georgia, 3, 113, 157, 178
Germany, 140, 187
gerontology, 186
Gestalt, 27
gestation, 7, 23, 24, 26, 27, 29, 50, 58, 64, 65, 66, 72, 73, 76, 78, 79, 81, 102, 103, 114, 115, 118, 119, 120, 122, 123, 124, 154
gestational age, 19, 20, 21, 26, 29, 48, 50, 61, 66, 69, 71, 78, 114, 115, 117, 118, 122, 123, 126, 130, 148, 154, 167
gestational diabetes, 73, 77
gigantism, 29, 50
gingivae, 35
gland, 23
glaucoma, 33
global scale, 161
gluconeogenesis, 56
glucose, 62, 63, 72, 73, 75, 81, 89, 90
glycogen, 51, 56, 72
glycosaminoglycans, 139
God, 12
gonorrhea, 20
grades, 121

graffiti, 144, 147, 153
graph, 77
Greece, 177, 183
growth, 19, 20, 23, 30, 48, 72, 113, 115, 148, 149, 154, 163, 172, 181
guidance, 50, 165
guidelines, 15, 60, 78, 102, 171

H

hair, 24, 32, 40
hair loss, 32
hazards, 21, 161
head injury, 165
healing, 8
health care, 7, 10, 11, 31, 67, 80, 114, 133, 152, 162, 164, 166, 173, 182
health care professionals, 10
health care system, 114, 152
health condition, 157, 160, 172
health researchers, 143
health risks, 144
health services, 159
health status, 157, 158
heart block, 21, 26
heart disease, 52
heart failure, 57
heart murmur, 19, 20, 52, 54, 63
heart rate, 27, 28, 37, 48, 52, 72, 104, 107, 108, 109
height, 41
hematology, 57
hematomas, 38
hemihypertrophy, 33
hemoglobin, 57, 58
hemoglobinopathies, 58
hemophilia, 137
hemorrhage, 29, 38, 53, 54, 56, 58, 121, 124
hemostasis, 136
hemothorax, 52
hepatitis, 22, 23, 60
hepatitis a, 23, 60
hepatocytes, 59
hepatomegaly, 59
hepatosplenomegaly, 22

hernia, 25
heroism, 14
hiatal hernia, 55
high school, 150, 174
history, 14, 19, 20, 21, 50, 51, 52, 55, 60, 61, 63, 71, 74, 76, 77, 84, 94, 99, 103, 166
HIV, 20, 23, 61, 132, 133, 135, 137, 140, 141, 142, 159, 164, 172, 174
HIV/AIDS, 159, 164, 172
home deliveries, 5
home ownership, 150
homelessness, 21, 144
homeostasis, 81, 147, 148
homes, 87, 100, 125, 151, 152, 154, 157, 167
Hong Kong, 183, 187, 190
hopelessness, 148
hormone(s), 27, 37, 39, 148, 149
hospital deliveries, 5
hospitalization, 48, 67
host, 172
hotels, 161
House, 140, 173, 186
House of Representatives, 140
housing, 87, 143, 145, 146, 147, 152, 153, 156
HPA axis, 147
HPV, 134, 141
hue, 32, 58
human, 7, 20, 85, 93, 103, 119, 129, 132, 134, 141, 174, 178, 185, 188, 189, 191
human brain, 119, 129
human development, 174, 178, 185, 188, 189, 191
human genome, 93
human immunodeficiency virus, 20, 132
human papilloma virus, 134
Hunter, 9, 14
hyaline, 13, 14
hyaline membrane disease, 13
hydrocephalus, 22, 23, 61, 121
hydrocephaly, 25
hydronephrosis, 23
hydrops, 22, 25, 26, 38, 57

hygiene, 6, 131, 134, 135
hyperactivity, 123, 130, 166
hyperbilirubinemia, 58, 59, 64, 70, 77, 79, 81
hyperglycemia, 50
hyperinsulinism, 56
hypernatremia, 56
hypertelorism, 24, 32
hypertension, 21, 24, 29, 50, 72, 116, 117, 163, 169, 172
hyperthermia, 24, 51, 53, 63
hypertrophy, 21, 50
hypoglycemia, 24, 29, 39, 51, 53, 56, 72, 73, 74
hyponatremia, 24
hypoparathyroidism, 56
hypoplasia, 24, 40
hypospadias, 39, 137, 139
hypotension, 75, 104, 109
hypothalamus, 147
hypothermia, 10, 19, 20, 51, 54, 63, 73
hypothesis, 135
hypothyroidism, 21, 24, 35, 37, 38, 56, 58, 61, 91, 92, 98, 100
hypovolemic shock, 110
hypoxia, 27, 30, 50, 54, 70, 104

I

ideology, 12, 13
illusion, 34
image, 40
immersion, 8
immune system, 115, 146, 169
immunodeficiency, 30
improvements, 6, 7
impulses, 119
in utero, 102, 103
incarceration, 164
incidence, 52, 67, 70, 73, 85, 108, 114, 134, 142, 145, 166
income, 116, 125, 128, 146, 163, 166, 169
incompatibility, 58
incubator, 4, 6
India, 173, 177, 183
individual perception, 145
individuals, 84, 85, 91, 95, 96, 97, 110, 148, 157, 158, 159, 160, 161, 172, 182
induction, 136
industrial revolution, 160
industrialization, 160
industries, 163
industry(s), 5, 133, 154, 161, 163
infant care, 4, 6
infant mortality, 5, 12, 13, 158, 168
infarction, 29, 50, 54
infection, 6, 7, 10, 20, 22, 29, 31, 33, 35, 50, 52, 56, 57, 59, 60, 61, 74, 75, 76, 116, 134, 135, 141, 142
infestations, 21
inflammation, 51, 169
inflation, 10
informed consent, 83, 94, 95, 97
infrastructure, 158
inguinal, 40
inhibition, 84
inhibitor, 59
initiation, 10, 91
injections, 165
injury(s), 29, 35, 53, 115, 120, 129, 139, 140, 158, 162, 181
innovator, 6
insecurity, 166
institutions, 48, 136, 149, 159
insulation, 119, 147
insulin, 50, 73
integration, 190
integrity, 70, 117, 151
intellectual disabilities, 174
intelligence, 145
intelligence tests, 145
intensive care unit, 7, 118, 127
internal processes, 148
internally displaced, 173
interneurons, 120
internship, 178
intervention, 35, 39, 57, 59, 60, 79, 115, 126, 128, 130, 142, 152, 156, 164
intervention strategies, 152
intestinal obstruction, 38, 39, 49

intestinal perforation, 24
intrauterine growth retardation, 23, 117, 148, 149
intravenously, 76
investment, 169
ipsilateral, 32, 34, 46
iris, 33
irritability, 19, 20, 29, 52, 53, 56, 63, 73, 75
IRT, 98
ischemia, 104
Israel, x, 3, 178, 183, 185, 186, 188, 190, 191
issues, 5, 50, 80, 83, 94, 131, 141, 182, 189, 190, 191

J

jaundice, 19, 20, 21, 22, 29, 33, 36, 38, 49, 51, 57, 58, 59, 60, 63, 75, 77, 118
jurisdiction, 140

K

Kenya, 142
kidney(s), 38, 104
kill, 11, 12
Kosovo, 159, 173

L

lack of opportunities, 144
lactation, 6, 77
landscape, 94, 127
laryngoscope, 10
larynx, 9
latency, 97
later life, 155
Latin America, 171
laws, 172
leadership, 155, 171
leakage, 38
learning, 11, 85, 118, 123, 124, 127, 129, 161, 164, 165, 166
learning disabilities, 124, 166

lecithin, 27
left atrium, 103
left ventricle, 103
legs, 41, 46, 47
lens, 33
lesions, 24, 32, 35, 36, 53, 120, 132
lethargy, 19, 20, 24, 37, 51, 52, 53, 54, 57, 73, 75, 79
life expectancy, 11, 166, 168
lifetime, 15
light, 33, 43, 92, 127, 133
liver, 58, 59
living conditions, 148, 160
loans, 152
local anesthetic, 136, 137
love, 11
low birthweight, 155, 156
low risk, 53, 115, 134
lumbar puncture, 53, 76
lung disease, 123
lying, 48
lymph, 36, 52
lymph node, 36

M

magnetic resonance, 124
magnetic resonance imaging, 124
magnitude, 161
majority, 67, 84, 92, 97, 148, 150
malaria, 159, 170
malnutrition, 30, 50, 92, 159
man, 5, 14, 143, 144
management, 6, 7, 8, 19, 53, 64, 73, 74, 80, 92, 94, 114, 115, 117, 118, 119, 127
manufacturing, 163
Marfan syndrome, 33
marketing, 92
marriage, 6
mass, 33, 36, 38, 62, 86, 97, 100
mass spectrometry, 86
mastitis, 37
maternal smoking, 154
maternal-fetal care, 4
maternity hospitals, 4

matrix, 146
matter, 91, 127
measurement(s), 10, 29, 66, 77, 88, 154
meconium, 10, 24, 38, 40, 49, 52, 55, 61,
 71, 104, 107
media, 172
Medicaid, 87, 156, 164
medical, 4, 11, 20, 21, 31, 66, 67, 76, 88,
 93, 94, 96, 97, 100, 117, 118, 119, 124,
 127, 131, 132, 133, 134, 136, 140, 141,
 152, 158, 166, 172, 178, 181, 182, 183,
 190
medical care, 11, 76, 94, 190
medical history, 21, 136
medical reason, 141
medication, 22, 35, 117, 166, 174
medicine, 4, 6, 8, 11, 12, 13, 79, 94, 96,
 129, 177, 181, 182, 188, 189
medulla, 54
mellitus, 72
membership, 177
membranes, 74, 76, 115
memory, 105
meningitis, 21, 22, 53, 56, 63
mental health, 117, 146, 162, 164
mentor, 7, 171
mentoring, 152
mentorship, 153
Mercury, 24, 161, 173
messages, 119
meta-analysis, 130, 155
Metabolic, 24, 29, 53, 54
metabolic acidosis, 28, 37, 53, 109
metabolic disorder(s), 27, 56, 85, 86
metabolism, 51, 53, 56
metastatic disease, 38
methemoglobinemia, 54
microcephaly, 22, 24
military, 88, 163
miosis, 33
misconceptions, 6
mission, 185
modern society, 11
modifications, 94, 96
modus operandi, 10

moisture, 147
mold, 144, 146, 164
morbidity, 67, 70, 80, 123, 154, 159, 170
morphology, 34
mortality, 11, 15, 67, 80, 154, 158, 159,
 162, 164, 170, 173
mortality rate, 11, 158, 173
Moses, 142
mosquitoes, 170
MRI, 61, 62, 124, 127
mucous membrane, 22
multiple factors, 162
murmur, 37, 54, 62
muscles, 38, 70, 104
muscular dystrophy, 97
musculoskeletal, 183
mutations, 87
mutilation, 140
mutual respect, 144
myasthenia gravis, 21
myelin, 119
myocarditis, 21, 22
myocardium, 109

N

nares, 35, 62
National Academy of Sciences, 102
national policy, 93
National Research Council, 155
national strategy, 12
natural disaster, 165
neglect, 165
neighborhood characteristics, 150
neonatal sepsis, 76
neonates, 67, 123, 124, 129, 139
nephrosis, 23
nerve, 54
nervous system, 70, 114
neurobiology, 155
neuroblastoma, 38
neurodevelopmental disorders, 172, 182
neurogenic bladder, 38
neuroimaging, 127
neurons, 119, 120

neurotoxicity, 77
neutral, 71
neutropenia, 21
New South Wales, 129
New Zealand, 6
newborn care, 5, 6, 15, 52
next generation, 171, 188
nicotine, 149
Nigeria, 161, 162, 173
Nobel Prize, 179
North America, 13, 14, 182
Norway, 187
NRP, 102, 105, 109, 110
nuclear family, 168
nurses, 16
nursing, 49, 119
nutrients, 149
nutrition, 49, 98, 117, 127, 170
nystagmus, 33

O

obesity, 29, 72, 151, 156, 163, 169, 173, 174, 190
obstacles, 162
obstetrician, 4, 5, 8, 9, 14
obstruction, 23, 25, 31, 35, 38, 52, 55, 63, 134
oligodendrocytes, 120
one dimension, 150
opacity, 33
operations, 161, 163
ophthalmia neonatorum, 5, 12
ophthalmologist, 6
opiates, 109
opportunism, 13
opportunities, 126, 144, 145, 160, 161, 162, 163
opt out, 97
optical density, 27
optimism, 118, 148
oral antibiotic(s), 138
organ(s), 38, 102, 104, 108, 115, 118, 127, 163
organism, 147

orthopedic surgeon, 5
osteogenesis imperfecta, 33, 40
otoacoustic emissions, 34, 85
outpatient, 79
overlap, 93
ownership, 152
ox, 62, 102, 103
oxidation, 98
oxygen, 6, 10, 15, 54, 71, 102, 103, 104, 108, 109, 118
oxygen consumption, 71

P

Pacific, 67
pain, 43, 141
palate, 35, 62
pallor, 19, 20, 51, 53, 57, 73
palpation, 20, 36
pancreas, 73
parallel, 103, 140
paralysis, 5, 29, 54
parasites, 21
parental support, 165
parenthood, 191
parents, 50, 84, 90, 96, 97, 118, 125, 127, 141, 164, 165, 190
patent ductus arteriosus, 54
paternalism, 94
pathogenesis, 130
pathogens, 76, 135
pathology, 38
pathophysiological, 120
pathophysiology, 127
pathways, 119, 120, 144, 145, 146, 147, 151
patient care, 137
pediatrician(s), 5, 6, 7, 10, 23, 27, 100, 164, 177, 181
pedigree, 95
peer review, 171
penetrance, 97
penicillin, 6, 13
penis, 39, 132, 134, 135, 137
percentile, 49
perfusion, 75, 104, 109, 110

perinatal, 4, 6, 11, 12, 13, 15, 16, 71, 81, 122, 123, 129, 130
perinatology, 4, 12
perineum, 39
peripheral neuropathy, 24
peritonitis, 38, 39
permission, 75
petechiae, 75
pH, 63
pharynx, 37
phenylalanine, 84, 85, 92
phenylketonuria, 83, 99, 100
Philadelphia, 13, 64, 129
philtrum, 29, 35
phosphate, 56
phospholipids, 139
photophobia, 33
physical environment, 144, 159
physical features, 143, 150
physical health, 155
physical structure, 146
physicians, 102
Physiological, 147
physiological mechanisms, 148
physiology, 14, 102, 127, 166
pitch, 37, 56
placenta, 21, 50, 57, 58, 73, 102, 110
placenta previa, 110
placental abruption, 29, 116
plants, 162
platelet count, 76
platelets, 76
platform, 171
playing, 118
pleural effusion, 36
pneumonia, 22, 37, 52
pneumothorax, 9, 52
policy, 86, 94, 140, 141, 152, 188
policymakers, 143, 145, 152
political parties, 140
politics, 140
pollution, 153, 163, 172, 173
polycystic kidneys, 38
polycythemia, 21, 29
polydactyly, 40

polyhydramnios, 23, 50, 52, 55
polyuria, 25
population, 65, 66, 73, 81, 87, 90, 93, 117, 119, 129, 158, 161, 162, 163, 164, 166, 173
population group, 117, 158
positive relationship, 127
poverty, 147, 150, 161, 162, 163, 164, 166, 168, 169, 172, 174
precordium, 37
predictability, 165
preeclampsia, 115
pregnancy, ix, 19, 20, 22, 23, 27, 76, 107, 114, 115, 116, 117, 126, 127, 128, 145, 148, 149, 154, 155, 160, 164, 167, 169, 174
pregnant mothers, 4, 144, 152, 153
premature baby, 4
premature infant, 4, 7, 9, 15, 81, 108, 113, 114, 115, 117, 118, 120, 121, 124, 125, 126, 127, 129, 130, 164, 169
prematurity, 7, 67, 78, 98, 113, 114, 115, 116, 117, 118, 120, 121, 122, 123, 124, 125, 126, 128, 129, 130, 166
preparation, 44
prepuce, 132, 134
President, 6, 7, 100, 113, 157
preterm delivery, 147, 148, 149, 154
preterm infants, 65, 70, 72, 73, 77, 79, 80, 81, 120, 130
prevention, 10, 12, 13, 15, 75, 128, 130, 133, 138, 140, 142, 169, 174, 179
primary teeth, 35
principles, 4, 6, 11, 80, 98
private practice, 178
proband, 95
professionals, 102, 171, 186, 188
profit, 152
progesterone, 62
project, 15, 93, 94, 153, 170, 171
prophylaxis, 32, 33, 51, 76, 131, 132
prostaglandins, 52
protection, 5, 181
psychological distress, 148
psychopharmacology, 182

psychosocial factors, 154
psychosocial stress, 147
psychotropic medications, 166
pubis, 39
public assistance, 67
public health, 92, 145, 153, 154, 160, 164, 173, 178, 185, 186, 188, 189, 190
public policy, 96
public resources, 168
public service, 163, 185
puericulture movement, 4
pulmonary arteries, 103
pulmonary hypertension, 24, 52, 104
pulmonary vascular resistance, 103
pumps, 103
purpura, 22
pyloric stenosis, 55
pyridoxine, 56

Q

quality assurance, 94
quality control, 13, 93
quality of life, 144, 179
quality standards, 152

R

race, 6, 74, 75, 88, 97, 155, 162
radar, 88
rales, 37, 52
rash, 68
reactivity, 50
reality, 15, 116, 119, 168
recall, 8
recognition, 65, 125, 177
recommendations, 15, 65, 75, 76, 98, 141
recreation, 163
recreational, 163
recreational areas, 163
rectum, 8, 63
red blood cells, 110
reflexes, 44
Reform, 13

refugee camps, 159
Registry, 163
regression, 21, 41, 50
rehabilitation, 179, 185
reliability, 92, 98
relief, 55, 140
religion, 16, 162
renal failure, 56
repair, 38, 39, 138, 165
reproduction, 6
requirements, 171
researchers, 96, 150, 189
reserves, 51, 72
Residential, 150
resilience, 152
resistance, 40, 102
resources, 92, 113, 119, 124, 128, 146, 149, 152, 157, 158, 159, 160, 163, 182
respiration, 28, 35, 36, 70, 107
respirator, 13
respiratory distress syndrome, 71, 118
respiratory failure, 7
respiratory problems, 37
respiratory therapist, 102
response, 29, 33, 44, 45, 46, 47, 50, 54, 148
retardation, 72, 148, 149, 154
retinoblastoma, 33
retinopathy, 7, 108, 118
retirement, 14
RH, 142, 155
rhinitis, 35
rhonchi, 37, 52
rhythm, 37
rhythmicity, 50
right atrium, 103
right ventricle, 103
rights, 11
risk factors, 53, 70, 72, 74, 75, 76, 77, 78, 79, 116, 117, 130, 134, 149, 155
Royal Society, 14, 122
rubella, 6, 13, 20, 23
rural areas, 160

S

safety, 77, 153

salivary gland, 35

saturation, 52, 62, 108

scholarship, 177

school, 126, 130, 144, 145, 152, 163, 164, 165, 166, 172, 174, 188, 190

science, 15, 73, 84, 186

scoliosis, 40

scrotal, 39

scrotum, 39, 68

secretion, 37

security, 168

seizure, 24

self-concept, 148

self-worth, 151

Senate, 140

sensation, 42

sensing, 163

sensitivity, 85, 88, 89, 90, 99

sepsis, 20, 22, 51, 53, 54, 56, 57, 60, 63, 73, 74, 75, 76, 79, 81, 118, 123

septum, 103

serum, 49, 57, 77

services, 94, 117, 124, 126, 128, 130, 144, 146, 156, 160, 164, 166

SES, 125

sexual activity, 134, 135, 164

sexual health, 182

sexual orientation, 162

sexuality, 191

sexually transmitted diseases, 132, 164

shape, 31, 32, 34, 90, 157

showing, 105, 114, 134

sibling(s), 46, 47, 92

sickle cell, 50, 58

sickle cell anemia, 50

side effects, 166

signals, 148

signs, 41, 48, 52, 57, 60, 63, 67, 70, 75, 76, 94, 95, 124, 144

silver, 5

Singapore, 158, 182

sinuses, 34, 36, 40

skin, 22, 24, 34, 36, 38, 40, 59, 104, 107, 117, 135, 136, 137, 138, 139

skull fracture, 32

sleep apnea, 163

small intestine, 104

smoking, 134, 149, 155, 172

social activities, 150

social capital, 146, 149, 155, 156

social care, 4

social consequences, 127

social control, 147, 153

social environment, 144, 155, 159

social life, 149

social organization, 149, 155

social relations, 149

social relationships, 149

social services, 165

social status, 146

social structure, 159

social support, 149

society, 11, 85, 91, 94, 95, 127, 128, 160, 168, 169, 170, 186

socioeconomic status, 116, 117, 146, 162

solution, 5, 132

Somalia, 158

South Africa, 135, 158

South America, 161

SP, 130

specialists, 181

species, 11

spherocytosis, 58

sphincter, 55

spina bifida, 23, 40

spinal cord, 22

spine, 40, 46

stability, 117, 118, 149, 150

stabilization, 71

standard deviation, 29, 50, 121

state(s), 11, 27, 34, 43, 48, 73, 75, 83, 85, 86, 87, 90, 91, 95, 98, 130, 148, 166, 168

statistics, 128, 150, 158

stenosis, 52, 55, 139

sternocleidomastoid, 36

sternum, 77

steroids, 141

stethoscope, 37
stigma, 95, 96
stimulation, 105, 164
stock, 87
stomach, 10, 52, 55
storage, 35
street drugs, 21
stress, 11, 27, 53, 98, 113, 117, 144, 146, 147, 148, 149, 150, 151, 153, 154, 155, 161, 165, 169, 174
stress factors, 117
stress response, 148, 169
stress test, 27
stressful life events, 155
stressors, 147, 148, 149, 152
stretching, 39
stridor, 37, 52
stroke, 48
structure, 59, 144, 172
substance abuse, 21, 109, 117, 144, 155, 164, 166, 172
substrate, 168
sudden infant death syndrome, 24, 67
Sun, 189, 190
supraventricular tachycardia, 26
surface area, 50
surfactant, 7, 14, 70, 108, 118
surfactant administration, 7
surveillance, 96
survival, 44, 113, 114, 118, 123, 127, 128, 130
survivors, 123, 129
susceptibility, 159
sustainability, 173
suture, 32, 138
sweat, 62
Sweden, 93, 122, 158, 187
symmetry, 35
symptoms, 51, 52, 56, 58, 75, 94, 95, 153
syndrome, 6, 21, 23, 24, 29, 31, 34, 35, 36, 37, 38, 41, 50, 53, 56, 57, 58, 60, 62, 71, 119, 165
synthesis, 139
syphilis, 4, 20, 35

T

tachycardia, 24
tachypnea, 19, 20, 28, 37, 48, 51, 52, 53, 54, 57, 63, 70, 73
target, 86, 94, 152
target population, 94
Task Force, 141
tax base, 163
Tay-Sachs disease, 87, 95, 97
techniques, 10, 80, 99, 127, 131, 136, 138
technology(s), 4, 92, 100, 113, 114, 115, 127, 160
teenage girls, 116
teeth, 23, 35
temperature, 4, 7, 19, 20, 48, 51, 52, 71, 75, 76, 79, 117, 124, 147
tenants, 149
tension, 138, 158
tenure, 149
test scores, 125
testicle, 62
testing, 19, 23, 85, 86, 87, 90, 92, 94, 96, 124
textbook(s), 5, 31, 48, 64, 102, 105, 178, 182
thalamus, 120
therapy, 13, 14, 23, 76, 77, 100, 103, 131, 138, 161
thinning, 68, 139
thorax, 47
threats, 162
thrombocytopenia, 21, 22, 23
thrombocytopenic purpura, 21
thrombosis, 29, 38
thyroid, 36, 57, 91, 98, 99
thyrotoxicosis, 21
tissue, 37, 109, 132, 138
Title V, 166
tobacco, 8, 21, 50, 117, 150, 166
tobacco smoke, 8
toddlers, 124
tones, 37, 52
tonic, 32, 56
torsion, 42, 137, 138

torticollis, 32, 36
toxicity, 159, 161
toxicology, 63
toxicology studies, 63
toxoplasmosis, 21, 61
trachea, 37, 107
tracks, 139
trade, 160
trainees, 107
training, 10, 102, 110, 136, 186
traits, 34, 50
transfer payments, 150
transformation, 135, 181
transfusion, 13, 25, 29
transition period, 28
translation, 12
transmission, 20, 21, 119, 135, 141, 164
transportation, 152
trauma, 5, 31, 52, 56, 122
treaties, 172
treatment, 6, 13, 15, 21, 53, 65, 67, 85, 87,
    91, 92, 93, 94, 98, 99, 138, 139, 155, 164
trial, 142
troubleshooting, 63
TSH, 61, 62, 91, 98
tuberculosis, 4, 20
tumor(s), 29, 33, 38, 39, 50
Turkey, 158
twins, 116, 154
twist, 138
tympanic membrane, 34
typhoid, 4
typhoid fever, 4
tyrosine, 62

U

ultrasonography, 66
ultrasound, 23, 40, 61, 62, 66, 123
umbilical cord, 62, 110
unconjugated bilirubin, 58
uniform, 86, 157
United Kingdom (UK), 13, 158, 187
United Nations (UN), 158, 159, 161, 169,
    173

United States, 3, 4, 5, 12, 16, 19, 65, 67, 83,
    99, 101, 113, 114, 131, 153, 157, 158,
    173, 174, 178, 183
universities, 171
urban, 155, 156, 172
urban population, 155
urbanization, 160
urethra, 138, 139
uric acid, 49
urinalysis, 51
urinary tract, 20, 131, 134, 142
urinary tract infection, 20, 131, 134, 142
urine, 38, 49, 51, 58, 61, 87, 117
US Department of Health and Human
    Services, 173
uterus, 148

V

vaccine, 134, 141
vacuum, 107
valve, 103
vandalism, 144, 153
variables, 150, 151
variations, 137
varus, 42
vasculature, 102, 103
vasoconstriction, 109
vein, 29, 38, 109
ventilation, 7, 8, 9, 10, 14, 104, 108, 109,
    110, 118, 147
ventricle, 103
vessels, 38, 52, 68, 104, 109, 138
violence, 16, 162, 172, 174, 191
violent behavior, 164
violent crime, 155
viral infection, 51, 56
viruses, 53
vision, 33, 34
volvulus, 55
vomiting, 19, 20, 51, 52, 53, 54, 55, 56, 57,
    75
vulnerability, 98, 114, 115, 120, 121

W

walking, 47
war, 4, 5, 173
Washington, 81, 100, 155, 173, 174
waste, 159
water, 6, 8, 48, 49, 58, 163
weakness, 8, 21, 36, 41, 44
wealth, 146, 152
weapons, 163
web, 138
weight gain, 71
weight loss, 80
welfare, 6, 152, 179, 185
well-being, 27, 117, 127, 158, 160, 179
wet nurse, 4
wheezing, 37
white blood cell differential, 76

white matter, 120
windows, 145, 147, 166
withdrawal, 24, 50, 56
wood, 4
World Health Organization (WHO), 15, 140, 159, 161, 169, 173
World War I, 6, 163
worldwide, 134, 140, 158

X

x-rays, 62

Y

young adults, 99, 174, 182
young people, 190
young women, 164, 168